A Measure of Health

Charis Williams

Contents

Preface

To the reader,

This is to be your guide to navigate you through your weight loss journey. It will clear up the confusion and help you to see and understand weight loss and fitness the way it's supposed to be: naturally. No counting calories, no starving in between meals, and the most important of all, targeted weight loss.

Most people want to get rid of their belly fat, and that is what this book addresses. It helps you to take a closer look at your lifestyle so that you can identify the things that cause belly fat and eliminate or reduce them.

Basically, it's your belly fat handbook. When you want to lose the belly, you'll know everything you need to know to be able to lose it, and fast.

Taking a few tips from this book will help you lose belly fat, and taking all the tips will give you even better and faster results. Consider which changes you are willing and interested in making as you read through the book.

Wishing you success on your fitness journey.

Charis Williams

Chapter One

What is a healthy waist size?

W hen discussing belly fat, it's important to ask this question first:

What is a healthy waist size?

We first need to use a reliable health measure:

Waist-to-hip Ratio

Waist-to-hip ratio is what researchers often use to measure health risk. We know that certain waist sizes can be unhealthily large all by themselves, but it is more important to measure the bodily proportions in relation to one another. The hips are supposed to be larger/wider in proportion to the waist[1].

This type of shape is a physical indication of healthy muscles and bones, low inflammation, a healthy heart and liver, and other healthy organs in the body.

Cardiovascular Health Risk by Waist-Hip-Ratio	Female	Male
Low	0.80 and under	0.95 and under
Moderate	0.81-0.85	0.96-1.0
High	0.86 and up	1.0 and up

Some people think weight loss is only for those who are considered "fat" or overweight, but weight loss is necessary for both the people who are of normal weight as well as those who are obese. The goal is to make sure that the **proportions** of the body are healthy.

So what is a healthy waist size?

Waist divided by Hips = Waist-to-hip ratio (WHR)

Researchers use waist-to-hip ratio to measure health risk, and have identified a healthy WHR to be below 0.80 for women and below 0.90 for men[2].

Your waist-to-hip ratio is so important to monitor because research has found that for every 0.10 rise in our waist-to-hip ratio, we statistically raise our risk of death[3].

Now we know what a healthy WHR is, but there is a limit to how large one can allow their waist to get while remaining healthy at the same time. A waist size that is thought of by researchers to be healthy, is measured to be under 31 inches (80 cm) wide around the belly button for women, and under 37 inches (94 cm) for men[4].

Despite what each individual considers to be the ideal body shape, most of society today is seeing their waistlines expand, regardless of their efforts to lose weight. Between 1988 and 2000, women's waistlines expanded from 34.9 inches to 36.2 inches. And for men, from 37.5 inches to 38.8 inches[5]. Our waistlines have been collectively expanding over time.

Chapter Two

Why do our waistlines expand?

O ver time we've seen more changes in our waistlines happening much faster, with abdominal obesity rising from 46.4% in the year 2000 to 54.2% in the year 2012 [6]. And in 2018, abdominal obesity was reported to be 67.33% of women and 49.73% of men [7]. At this rate we will all end up with it. So what's going on?

Our waists are not just cosmetic, they're a reflection of our health.

The size of our waists predict our natural deaths. One study revealed that despite our different Body Mass Indexes, if we have a disproportionately larger waist, we have a 25% increased risk of death regardless of how old we are [8]. This isn't entirely about looks, basically, due to the fact that the waist is part of the human body, it serves as a good indicator to help us tell if we're healthy. Our health changes over time and in response to what we do and what we're surrounded by, and because our waists are a part of our body, our level of health is demonstrated by our waists.

There are two types of belly fat:

1. Visceral (wraps around the organs) and

2. Subcutaneous - the fat you can grab, the fat right under the skin.

Visceral fat has been recognized as a major risk factor for heart disease, cancer, cerebrovascular disease, and diabetes. Lowering belly fat tends to reverse the disease state of people who have these conditions, and increasing belly fat tends to push people into these disease states.

This is regardless of how "skinny" a person may be. Belly fat is something that is important to wield your control over, and achieving an hourglass figure isn't just a look or a fashion to have, it's a healthy lifestyle that results in a better quality of life.

Belly fat is an issue that is even seen in our bloodwork:

- High blood pressure,

- Issues disrupting proper endothelial function,

- Increasing/elevated triglycerides,

- High LDL "bad" cholesterol,

- Low HDL "good" cholesterol,

- Digestive issues,

- Heart/circulation issues, and

- Metabolic issues (for example glucose and insulin malfunctions)

Having a larger waist can even mean that a person is twice as likely to die when they get to be 50 or older [9].

An important thing to get under control is your triglycerides. Researchers have a word they use to describe wide waists, the "hypertriglyceridemic" waist is 90 cm or a 35 inch waist in men and 85 cm or a 33.4 inch waist in women.

Male	Female
90 cm or 35 in	85 cm or 33.4 in

By the time a person is identified as having a hypertriglyceridemic waist, they have a higher risk of [10]:

- High blood pressure,

- Increased inflammation,

- Low good cholesterol,

- More dangerous sizes of bad cholesterol, and

- Coronary artery disease

This waist size is also particularly associated with having a higher risk of developing coronary artery disease [11].

Belly fat is a major sign of inflammation in the body. People with more belly fat have been found to have more signals of inflammation [12]:

- C-reactive protein,

- Compliment C3,

- Interleukin-6,

- Retinol binding protein-4,

- Tumor necrosis factor A,

- Amyloid A, and

- White blood cell counts

Belly fat is actually a visual sign of someone's lifestyle and their possibility of developing certain health problems in the future. Belly fat shows that there are possible underlying issues with insulin sensitivity, glucose, and fatty acid metabolism [13]. This means that if you want to get rid of toxic belly fat, you *have to* embrace a safe, health promoting lifestyle. *There is no other option or shortcut.*

Chapter Three

Why is hip size important?

It's also important to mention how important hip size is. In order to have an hourglass figure, a small waist is necessary, BUT proportionately larger gluteal muscles and gluteal fat is just as important. The fat in our glutes is healthy and protective. This type of fat is a sign that the body has a healthy lipid and glucose profile, and also less chance of cardiovascular and metabolic malfunction [14].

People with larger hips have been found to experience more satisfaction after eating and also less inflammation in their bodies. In fact, it has been shown that the more inflammation we cause in our bodies, the more our glutes get smaller [15].

This is where your lifestyle changes everything, because it has been proven that as we lose our gluteofemoral fat and muscles, we begin to develop metabolic and cardiovascular problems [16].

	Large Waist	Small Waist
Small Thighs	More likely to have unhealthy glucose levels	Somewhere in-between
Larger Thighs	Somewhere in-between	Less likely to have unhealthy glucose levels

Regarding glucose alone, women who have large waists and small thighs are especially in danger of having unhealthy glucose levels as compared to women with smaller waists and larger thighs [17]. Glucose levels are so important because they can represent a healthy metabolism but can also represent the beginning of a downward spiral when it comes to Type II diabetes depending on what those levels are. Abdominal obesity is a marker of elevated diabetes risk [18].

Elevated fasting glucose, also known as prediabetes, is the first small sign from your lab work that something is metabolically abnormal, and this state of health is visibly shown on our bodies.

So if there's one thing that is important to remember for your life decisions, know that our waists are a reflection of our health.

There's a lifestyle that creates a V shape or hourglass figure, all it takes is adopting that lifestyle to see the results.

Chapter Four

Should I be concerned with calories?

C alories are unnecessary to monitor when it comes to the waist. Weight loss is supposed to be more of an intuitive and natural process, it is not necessary and it is also stress-provoking to starve yourself or worry and obsess over calories. Focusing on calories can actually result in you developing *more* belly fat, so depriving yourself of food is not worth the effort. However there is an important key to keep in mind.

Calories are not just calories.

Certain calories are bad calories while other calories are good calories. When deciding on food to eat, don't get caught up watching your calories because it can leave you eating the wrong *types* of food that increase inflammation, make you feel *more hunger* and *cause fat to develop* in your stomach area.

If you follow a calorie-restricted diet, a calorie from an Oreo cookie and a calorie from a carrot are guaranteed to go in two different places. And I'm sure you can guess where the Oreo calorie will go. A few potato chips may be low in calories, but they specifically pack fat within the belly. Science is still in the process of discovering how the body works and how nutrition affects our genes and our body fat distribution, so when choosing healthy food items to eat, remember that calories are not the total answer.

So that brings me to the next point, if certain types of food have bad calories and other types have good calories, then how can you tell which is bad and which is good? Find out if the food causes inflammation.

The types of food that have <u>bad</u> calories are the types of food that <u>cause inflammation</u> on a cellular level in the body. When the body is inflamed, belly fat develops.

Inflammation ——— >> Belly Fat

Many research articles prove the connection between belly fat and inflammation. Belly fat is a sign of inflammation in the body even in people who are not overweight [19].

Research shows that those with abdominal fat exhibit 53% higher C-reactive protein levels, 30% higher Tumor Necrosis Factor A (TNF-a) levels, 26% Amyloid A levels, 17% higher white blood cell counts and 42% higher Interleukin-6 (IL-6) levels [2021].

Talk about inflammation!

So getting rid of belly fat is really a battle to lower the total inflammation levels in your body. But that isn't all there is to a bad calorie...

A bad calorie is also bad because it <u>lacks nutrition</u>. This may seem counterintuitive to the too common belief that when you're overweight it means you eat too much, but that isn't true. In fact, belly fat is a sign of ***malnutrition***.

A person who has too much belly fat is more likely to have any number of vitamin deficiencies including[222324252627282930]:

All fat-soluble vitamins:

- Vitamin A

- Vitamin D

- Vitamin E

- Vitamin K

Also...

- Vitamin C

- Beta-carotene and other carotenoids

- Folate

- Magnesium

- Thiamin

- Selenium

- Vitamin

- B12

- Calcium

This doesn't mean you should run to your nearest supplement store because supplements are <u>not as effective</u> as eating the actual food. Some supplements have been found to be synthetic and harmful, with negative effects, while the actual food has no negative effect. Supplements only provide one nutrient at a time, while *whole* unprocessed foods provide multiple nutrients at once without having to swallow pills or introduce anything synthetic into the body. Focus on getting nutrients primarily from **food** sources.

Nutrition is extremely important. Research confirms that people who are *obese* are deficient in *most* vitamins [31]. Obesity really isn't an issue of overeating as much as it is an issue of eating the wrong *types* of food - the food that is empty of nutrients, the food that causes bad health.

Obese people are also more likely to have less antioxidants in their bodies, antioxidants that are commonly found in nuts, citrus fruit, and yellow and orange vegetables like carrots and sweet potatoes.

The nutrients that play a helpful role in our metabolism and that prevent the development of fat in our bodies are less prevalent in obese people: Carotenoids, Vitamin E, Vitamin C, zinc, magnesium, and selenium [32].

There are studies that verify that people with metabolic issues are missing the proper amounts of vitamins A, D, E, and carotenoids [33]. When preventing metabolic issues (and losing body fat), it's important to make sure your body has the tools it needs to run properly and efficiently. Our bodies need the *right* type of fuel. This isn't just a matter of "dieting" and restricting yourself, this is a matter of getting *proper nutrition*.

So you may be wondering which came first, the metabolic issues or the nutritional deficiencies? Well, the nutritional deficiency came first: Children who start out life with nutritional deficiencies are more likely to become obese later in life [34]. Just imagine, years and years of eating food that isn't truly made to be consumed by the body. Processed food is not real food and that has its effects.

Between 15-29% of obese patients seeking bariatric surgery were deficient in the vitamin Thiamin [35]. That's a large percentage of obese people who are *deficient* in a vitamin, and this is only *one* of the vitamins listed earlier.

You may have heard of weight loss supplements like canthaxanthin or astaxanthin. Why are these supplements so popular and why do they work for so many people? Well as it turns out, they are *vitamins*: carotenoids. And a large waist size is a sign of a carotenoid deficiency [36].

Women with larger waists were found to have low levels of certain carotenoids [37]:

- canthaxanthin,

- alpha-carotene, and

- beta-carotene

Sometimes it isn't dietary though. Sometimes we simply aren't getting enough sun.

One study found that about 35% of obese people have Vitamin D deficiency while 24% of overweight people were deficient in Vitamin D [38]. It appears as though the more a person becomes deficient, the more body fat they end up with.

So it's time that we start viewing fat as a sign of *deficiency* rather than it being a sign of *overindulgence*.

Now that we've established that, it's important to remember <u>not to</u> ignore your body's hunger signals. The human body experiences hunger when it notices a need for nutrients. Nutritious food that doesn't add to belly fat is so compatible with our bodies on a biological level and therefore is nothing to be afraid of.

Our bodies were designed to process basic food, not processed food. Processed food does not satisfy our nutritional needs: the more processed a food item is, the less variety of nutrients it has.

When there are less nutrients, our bodies experience hunger *more intensely*, we like to call this hunger "craving," but that's because we typically we find ourselves giving in and eating food that causes weight gain.

Eating too much of an item that isn't nutritious is basically *robbing* our bodies of nutrients because the body has to *process* the food, and continue functioning as normal, <u>without the nutrients it needs</u>.

When your nutrient needs haven't been satisfied, the body will use hunger signals to remind you to eat. What happens when we eat processed food is that the body will recognize that it was tricked, and then it will become hungry again. It's the beginning of a continuous downward spiral unless some dietary changes are made for a lengthy amount of time to heal.

Food from nature is *biologically compatible* with our bodies. The less processed food is, the more *freely* you can eat of it, because it's satisfying to the body. That's why its important to emphasize eating the <u>right type</u> of food.

Our bodies are highly responsive to healthy food. It's nearly impossible to eat too much of it. The satiety hormone works ideally with healthy food, letting us know that we are no longer hungry in a timely manner that prevents us from overeating. Eating is supposed to be a natural process. Not a calorie-counting, weighing on a scale, and portion size measuring process.

Resisting hunger urges is dangerous territory because **hunger has a biological purpose**. Hunger is when our bodies are requesting nutrients. It isn't just because the food tastes or smells good, it's because our bodies need the nutrition. When we eat unhealthy food, more often than not, hunger comes again soon afterwards. The body didn't get what it wanted. The good news is that when we eat healthy food, we will be satisfied for much longer, because the body got what it wanted: nutrients.

So give your body what it wants so that it can work for you and make your life easier. <u>No fad diet and no amount of exercise will work if a deficiency is the cause of your belly fat.</u> Healthy-sized waists have less nutrient deficiencies, so make sure to focus on getting your nutrients!

Now if you're like most people you may be thinking that you're already eating in a pretty healthy way, but there are some special details that most people are unaware and uninformed of. We are going to go into much more detail about how to get your lifestyle on point so that you can be on track to get rid of your belly fat.

Chapter Five

Why fruits and veggies are not optional

A nything you can do to lower your chance of developing these diseases results in a smaller waist [394041]:

- Heart disease (including CAD, CHD, CVD)

- Cancer

- Type II Diabetes

- Metabolic Syndrome

- Elevated Glucose Levels aka prediabetes

- Hypertension

- Kidney disorders

- High triglycerides

- High cholesterol levels

- Inflammation/pain

- PCOS or other hormone imbalance

- Obesity

- Non-Alcoholic and Alcoholic Fatty Liver Disease

Think about it like this: each organ in your body needs to function. If your body is being fed fake food, it will not work at its best, at best it will be sluggish.

When tackling this issue with the goal of lowering your risk of these diseases, you have to focus on the things that you can control. That means, if there are any lifestyle changes that you *can* make to reduce your risk of these diseases, that's what you need to focus on and care about. Don't focus on the contributing factors that you cannot control.

Eat lots of veggies and fruit. They're rich in fiber and nutrients. Fiber and nutrient-rich food help result in the loss of belly fat. Raw fruits, veggies, and mushrooms have natural digestive enzymes in them so that instead of *causing issues* during digestion, they *help* to digest themselves.

Each fruit that you eat per day reduces the risk of heart disease by 5% and each vegetable reduces the risk of heart disease by 4%. Fruits and vegetables reverse inflammation in the body. Just one serving of green leafy vegetables per day reduces your risk of developing Type II Diabetes [42].

Most people understand that drinking juice isn't a good idea if you want to prevent diabetes (because it spikes insulin) but nothing is wrong with eating fruit. Many people fear fruit because it has natural sugars. But research informs us that green leafy vegetables and fruit actually lower the risk of diabetes [43]. The sugar in fruit is not the same as table sugar.

There's no need to be afraid of fruit. Fruit can help prevent diabetes and metabolic health issues. If a person were to eat fruit 3 times per day, their risk of diabetes still won't increase [44].

The sugar in fruit is *time-release*. It's in nature's perfect package, with all the other important vitamins, fiber, and minerals that our bodies need. Fruit protects the health of the metabolism. Ultimately when you deprive your body of fruit, you're removing a type of food that actually **prevents** diabetes.

Let's go a little more in-depth though:

Fruits <u>and</u> vegetables on average lower *all-cause mortality* by 5% for each serving. For vegetables you get a risk reduction of 5% and for fruit 6% [45][46]

The benefits are especially impactful for preventing cardiovascular disease.

<u>1 fruit per day</u>

6% reduced risk cardiovascular disease

<u>5 fruit per day</u>

30% reduced risk of *all-cause mortality*

After that, the risk-lowering effect of fruit goes away and it just becomes <u>neutral</u>. So sadly, eating 20 fruit a day won't make you immortal.

Eating a diet with unprocessed, whole vegetables, fruit, legumes, fish, poultry, and whole grains (also known as a "prudent diet") results in a 28% lower risk of cardiovascular death, and 17% lower risk of all types of death [47]. And we can do better than the prudent diet, it's just a matter of identifying the types of food that increase our mortality and lessen the chance of disease and inflammation.

What does fruit do for the body? Research has shown that fruit is an ultimate waist-slimmer and it also preserves the muscles in the glutes [48]. Its high nutrient content has special effects in the body that have been proven to result in more of an hourglass figure. This is what fruit does. Fruit is nature's highest source of potassium. It reduces belly fat, makes the waist smaller, and provides valuable nutrients and antioxidants.

Fruit that is rich in potassium actually has the effect of preserving muscle or lean body mass. Researchers measure how much potassium is being excreted or released from our urine because it shows how much potassium people eat in their diets. Those who eat more potassium-rich food have more muscle than those who don't eat as much potassium-rich food [49]. Fruit is beneficial for muscle health because it is nature's greatest source of potassium. Remember it's important to have lean body mass because it is a major part of our metabolism and it contributes to our hip circumference. Muscles also consume a lot of energy and are useful for fat loss because muscle uses fat for fuel.

Fruit has a lot of benefits but vegetables do too. Eating almost any vegetable helps lower inflammation in the body resulting in a smaller waist.

Green leafy vegetables are rich in phytonutrients. Phytonutrients are disease-preventing agents that are found in large amounts within plants. Phytonutrients help to reduce the risk of type II diabetes, high blood pressure, arthritis, and high cholesterol, and they help to make the waist smaller [50].

Green leafy vegetables as well as root vegetables help to prevent diabetes. Eating more root vegetables alone can reduce the risk of getting diabetes by 13% [51].

Carotenoids are found primarily in red, orange, and yellow fruits and vegetables. They help to prevent visceral belly fat [52]. They're so productive at getting rid of visceral fat, that supplementation with mixed carotenoids has been shown to make the waist smaller and lower overall body fat percentage [53].

Carotenoids are better absorbed when eaten with a dietary source of fat, because they are a *fat-soluble vitamin*. Make sure to include nuts, seeds, and avocados with your meals to help with the absorption of carotenoids from items like carrots and sweet potatoes.

There are certain carotenoids that people with larger waists don't have enough of: Canthaxanthin, beta-carotene, and alpha-carotene. Dark green vegetables, yellow-orange and red-orange vegetables, algae and even some mushrooms have these carotenoids in them.

Belly fat is widely known to be largely a dietary issue, but most of the time we think of it as an issue of "eating too much" rather than "eating too little." Belly fat can be caused by what you're NOT getting, not always by what you're getting. There are certain food items that have been shown to slim the waist, that are not commonly eaten in Western societies. The fact is that a lot of people who struggle with belly fat also don't get enough seaweed in their diets.

Seaweed is a sea vegetable that is high in iodine and carotenoids, both of which are necessary for having a healthy waist size. Seaweed has been shown to improve iodine status in women who don't have enough iodine [54]. The natural iodine from seaweed is essential for a healthy waist and a healthy metabolism.

One of the carotenoids that is found in seaweed is called fucoxanthin. When participants in a study took 3 MG of fucoxanthin daily for 4 weeks, they ended up losing some abdominal fat and decreasing their overall body weight [55].

Seaweed even counteracts the negative effects of a high (simple) carb and high (unhealthy) fat diet. Typically these diets result in a deterioration of health and significant gains in body fat, but when they studied rats on the diet while supplementing them with seaweed, they lost a significant amount of body fat (24% to be exact), and a reduction in triglycerides, blood pressure, and insulin levels! They also had better insulin and glucose sensitivity [56]. It's as though their diet didn't matter at all. If seaweed isn't a part of your diet yet, it may be truly beneficial for you. Consider how your body has been going years without a regular source of sea vegetables in your diet. Maybe your body was wanting this all along!

It's amazing how we can feed our bodies terribly for years and yet we can stay alive. Our bodies have to prioritize what's most important and if that means you develop belly fat over time from not getting enough nutrients, then that's what the body will do. The body needs to maintain homeostasis. It's a small price to pay for the amount of abuse that we put our bodies through.

But now is healing time, regeneration time. Time to turn things around and give your body everything it has been missing. If you focus on health, your waistline will follow.

Dried Fruit

Dried fruit is also known to make the waist smaller as well as lower your overall body fat percentage [57]. Dried fruit can be used instead of sugar and syrup to sweeten things. It can be rehydrated and then placed in the blender when you're ready to add its sweetness and nutrients to a dish. Just soak it in some water for a couple hours or overnight.

People who eat dried fruit have smaller waists, less body fat, and more nutrients in their diet [58]. Dried fruit can be a great tool when you get those cravings for sweet food. Eating dried fruit is so helpful because it's guilt-free.

The vitamin C in fruit helps with regulating the appetite, improves blood vessel health in a dose-response fashion, ultimately resulting in a reduced risk of heart failure. [596061]. They measured vitamin C levels in blood plasma and found that when it went up 20 umol/L (micro moles per liter), the risk of heart failure decreased by 9% [62]. People who have lower amounts of vitamin C are more likely to get heart failure. This just shows how important and completely necessary it is to make sure you're getting a certain amount of fruit on a daily basis.

Now if you're like most people you may be thinking fruits and veggies are nasty or that they are difficult to eat, but if you give it between 4-6 weeks, your taste buds should adjust [63].

The sooner you get started with eating your fruits and vegetables, the better your health, your energy, and your confidence will be over time. Give yourself a chance, and do yourself this favor and challenge yourself to do it for the results.

Chapter Six

The truth about carbs and belly fat

It's important that we can finally get clear on how carbs affect our waistlines and our health. Knowing about carbs will empower you to eat a diet that is truly nourishing and well balanced, leaving you with improved endurance fitness and a healthy waist size. So let's get started:

As you know, type II diabetes and heart disease are diseases that typically develop after you acquire belly fat. Whole grains such as barley, wheat, oat groats, millet, or brown rice reduce the risk of these diseases but they have to be *whole grains*, not processed. That means, pay attention to details when checking your food. The bread in the store with "whole grains" typed on it is often a misleading labeling that is made to entice you, so it is important to check *ingredient* labels and/or make healthy whole recipes yourself.

When choosing a type of bread, the best bread to get is one that lists whole grains, and no sugar or any other unusual mystery ingredients. Make sure the ingredients list contains whole grains. Eating lots of whole grains helps to get rid of and prevent visceral belly fat.

Despite the fact that we're in the age of low carb dieting, the truth is that carbohydrates in their whole form are *exactly what we need* to prevent diseases like diabetes. Whole grains prevent diabetes in a *dose-response* fashion [64]. That means that the more whole grains someone eats, the less likely they are to develop diabetes. Basically, if whole grains were a pill that a person could take to prevent diabetes, you'd want to take it as much as possible because it's been proven to work.

Many people think that the best way to slim your waist is to go for a low carb diet, carbohydrates aren't evil. In fact, our bodies prefer carbohydrates because they are the **#1 energy source** for our cells [65]. Low carb diets can be effective in the short term, but over the long term, it can become dangerous (and tiring) to remain in a state of ketosis [66].

Now-a-days whole grains seem like a forgotten food. Most of the grains that we see are processed, including most types of pasta, rice, and wheat. What makes real whole grains different is that whole grains have all of the necessary parts of the grain: the endosperm, germ and bran. Whole grains have been pushed out by the low-carb diet trend, but whole grains were never the problem, in fact, they were part of the *solution*.

Refined grains were the problem. Refined grains and whole grains have opposite effects on our waistlines and on our health. Consumption of refined grains is associated with having a larger waist while consumption of whole grains is associated with having a smaller waist [67].

In fact, those who eat the *most* whole grains have actually been found to have smaller waist measurements.

Whole grains have a way of transforming the body from the inside out. As carbohydrates tend to do, they have a way of affecting your blood glucose. These carbohydrates improve our health instead of damaging it, though [68].

When people do whole grain interventions, their fasting glucose decreases (lowering their likelihood of developing pre-diabetes) and the bad, waist expanding, and health deteriorating LDL cholesterol decreases [69][70].

Whole grains have been shown to reduce the risk of developing type II diabetes [71].

And for constipation, whole grains help significantly. These healthy carbohydrates ferment in the gut, helping to feed and develop healthy gut bacteria and helping to make poop heavier so that it can come out faster and more easily [72].

Whole grains are also far more satisfying than refined grains, which makes them great for reducing cravings and overeating because they have a positive impact on appetite-related hormones [73].

Whole grains are especially great when it comes to losing belly fat:

1. <u>Whole grains burn belly fat.</u> Whole grain eaters have smaller waists than those who don't eat whole grains. It has been shown that people who have 3 servings of whole grains daily have less subcutaneous fat (fat under the skin) and 10% less visceral fat (fat surrounding the organs) than those who have no whole grains daily [74].

2. <u>Whole grains *prevent* weight gain, too.</u> Over an 8 year span, around 40 grams or 1 serving of brown rice per day is enough to result in 2.4 lb or 1.1 kg less weight gain. So basically that means that 1 serving of brown rice daily helps to prevent weight gain. **Keep in mind that most Americans gain about 2 pounds per year** [75].

3. <u>Whole grains assist with geriatric/elderly weight loss.</u> Some people think that because they're much older than the average person trying to lose weight, that they can't lose belly fat, but one study confirmed that in older adults, those who ate more whole grains had less abdominal fat, and this was **dose-dependent** [76]. This means that the more whole grains they consumed, the less abdominal fat they had.

So carbohydrates aren't all bad, remember the whole grain carbs, because they're absolutely essential to have in your diet if you want to prevent weight gain in the belly. Carbohydrates *are* good when they come from whole grains. Three servings of whole grains a day is a great daily goal regardless of what else you eat. It's especially important to continue eating whole grains like brown rice to help lessen the negative effects of cheat meals.

Examples of whole grains include:

- Hulled barley

- Oat groats

- Brown jasmine rice

- Millet

- Buckwheat, etc.

So remember, the size of our waists reflect the health of our heart and our overall metabolism.

Whole grains are so important that if you *don't* have them in your diet, you're increasing your risk of heart failure. This is why it's important to pay attention to the quality of your diet when working towards losing belly fat. Our focus should not always be about what we are supposed to avoid, our focus should also be on what foods/habits we need to integrate into our lives on a consistent basis.

Refined Grains

We've discussed complex carbohydrates but let's discuss the evil carbohydrate counterparts. *Simple* carbohydrates are a *major* problem.

Processed grains, also known as simple carbs, increase both visceral and subcutaneous fat. Beware of packaged items like bread, crackers, pasta, tortillas and even slightly processed grains like white rice and quick oats.

Refined grains have the opposite effect of whole grains, they make the waist larger. Refined grains tend to sabotage weight loss efforts, but a *little* dietary flexibility can be forgiven by the body. In fact, one study, oddly enough, showed that the *smallest waists* were among people who had <u>both</u> whole grains and refined grains in their daily diet: 3 servings whole grain, and 2 or less of refined [77].

Just remember that one study isn't enough to confirm that it's safe to eat refined grains in such a frequent quantity. Even if a person eats 3 servings of whole grains every day, eating 2 servings of refined grains everyday will probably have some accumulative effects over the course of say, 15 years. It isn't a risk worth taking consistently over time. Remember that refined carbs are to be minimized and avoided, so this research should be used to help provide some freedom while engaging in the occasional cheat meal, but not an excuse to lose all self control and spiral into unchartered research territory by committing to eating refined carbohydrates with your whole grains every day. Be the one who controls how many refined carbohydrates you eat, do not be controlled by the refined carbohydrates.

Eating whole grains helps to result in less hospitalizations and lower death rates, they lower LDL and other types of bad cholesterol, making the waist smaller. Make sure to prioritize whole grains and be consistent with eating them every single day.

A lot of people think it is necessary to stop eating or significantly reduce all carbohydrates in order to lose weight and become healthier. And yes, this weight loss method is proven to work, but that's because it removes the human body's primary and *preferred* source of energy: carbohydrates.

Complex carbohydrates actually help the body to get rid of belly fat *and* overall body fat.

Whole grains reduce the waist-expanding LDL

In order for the body to lose belly fat, LDL, the bad cholesterol, needs to be lowered. If your LDL levels are not right, it is more likely that you are carrying some belly fat on your body. Whole grains have been proven to improve these cholesterol levels resulting in study participants having smaller waists [78].

Whole Grains Prevent Muscle Loss

A lot of us don't realize it, but we're constantly losing muscle mass. As we age, as we sit in front of our TVs and sit at our desks, barely ever getting any exercise and then turning around and eating things that cause inflammation in our bodies. As we eat food that doesn't have enough nutrition for our muscles to thrive... over time we experience muscle loss.

Muscle burns fat. Muscle is a major part of our metabolism and the less muscle we have, the slower our metabolism is. Having leg/thigh/butt muscles is especially important. Having muscles is associated with the presence of fertility and good HDL cholesterol levels.

Whole grain cereals (not the polluted brands with sugar, preservatives, food dyes and heavy metals added to them) have been shown to genetically up regulate muscle hypertrophy (growth/anabolism) genes and down regulate muscle atrophy (breakdown/catabolism) genes [79].

That means that whole grains alter your genes to *promote* and assist with muscle growth. Whole grains positively impact our muscles.

Helps Reduce Insulin Resistance

Maybe you don't have diabetes and maybe you do, but even if you don't, this is important to know: Insulin resistance isn't something that happens only in people who have diabetes. Insulin resistance is associated with fatty liver, arteriosclerosis, acanthuses nigricans, skin tags, and reproductive abnormalities [80]. Consuming whole grains helps to reduce insulin resistance which indirectly reduces the risk of all of these health issues.

Whole grains are a metabolism healer: whole grains improve glucose tolerance, metabolic flexibility, and peripheral insulin sensitivity [81].

Simply adding whole grains to your diet can mean better overall health and as your health improves and you lower your risk of diabetes, your waist will get smaller [82].

Any natural food that improves glucose and insulin resistance is likely to help your waist get smaller.

In addition to the fact that research confirms this, I personally have found that when I eat whole grains at every meal, even if it isn't a healthy meal, I'm better able to keep the belly fat away. So give it a try yourself since it's been proven to help others.

Chapter Seven

Dietary fat and how it affects the waistline

S ome types of fat are waist-friendly and some types of fat are an enemy to your waist and to your overall health.

In life it's so easy to just go for a low fat or a high fat diet, without separating the different *types* of fat. When you don't know the difference between good fat and bad fat, your results will be murky. Some people will lose belly fat, while others will gain belly fat, so this is all about finding clarity, so that you can get real and consistently good results.

Fried food and the Waist

Most people know that fried food is unhealthy, but did you know frying with *any* oil can be bad for you?

Oil, mixed with the metal of the frying pan, and high heat, results in a creation of chemicals that are harmful to human health. As you know, hypertension, heart disease and diabetes are where an oversized belly can take you in the long run... so it's important to know that eating fried food can give you an oversized belly, and fast.

It's also important to mention that **oil is the fatty equivalent to sugar:** It provides little to no nutrients, yet is quite energy dense. This means that your body has to digest it while receiving no nutrients in return. It has to work while being given *inferior* fuel. Oil stresses the body, yet doesn't contribute very much to its health.

Fried food increases belly fat and the risk of hypertension because of the frying process.

Sadly, olive oil is not as healthy as it has been made out to be. Triglycerides, as I mentioned before, are waist expanding. And research confirms that ALL vegetable oils, whether they are fresh or have been deep-fried, cause triglycerides to increase in healthy people, and this study included olive oil [83].

Triglycerides are something that you want to keep under control and within normal range if you want to have a healthy waist size. Researchers have coined the term "hypertriglyceridemic waist" to identify people who have large waists, *because they tend to have high triglycerides.* The problem with olive oil research is that it is always compared to a worse food item, a worse oil or to conventional butter. The marketing that is found on their products and in news articles can say things like "olive oil reduces waist size" but that is only in comparison to other sources of processed fat that have already been found to increase the size of the waist. Obviously, in comparison to olive oil, many oils are worse, yet it's important to know that it's *best* to abandon cooking with *all* oils. If you want a healthy waist size, you need to have healthy blood vessels and a healthy heart, and increasing your triglycerides is not the path that leads to achieving healthy blood vessels and a healthy heart.

Thankfully unheated and unprocessed monounsaturated fats like from fresh avocados can be protective from the damage that fried food causes in the body [84].

Even cooking with coconut oil has been shown to have negative health effects because the negative effects happen when it has been heated, and are especially bad when the oil has been reused and reheated over and over again. These oils increase blood pressure and inflammation in the body [85].

It's so important to stay away from fried food at restaurants and to stop frying food at home - fried food significantly contributes to the risk of developing both type II diabetes and coronary artery disease [86]. The research seems to suggest that people who have other blood vessel problems also need to consider quitting fried food as well.

Fried food, while quite enjoyable to eat, increases your levels of cholesterol, and increases your risk of obesity, hypertension, type II diabetes, and coronary artery disease [8788].

Most of us don't initially see a problem with oil, but there's enough evidence to suggest that it isn't really healthy, after-all. As I stated earlier, oil is like sugar in fat form. It is mostly missing nutrients and yet it is in an extremely pure high dose. Cooking with oil has been shown to increase inflammation in the blood vessels, the same type of inflammation that has been linked to belly fat [899091].

And while oil may be better than conventional butter when it comes to the levels of unhealthy fat in the blood, a diet *with* oil still can't outperform a diet *without* any added oil. Cutting oil will benefit your health and speed up your belly fat loss results!

Fatty food in whole form (nuts/avocados) is naturally made to be consumed by the human body and it also comes with other synergistic nutrients that help the body to do its job.

The problem with unhealthy food items like oil is that it hardly gives, it mostly takes. The body needs food and nutrients for fuel, and oil is not a good source of nutrients. If the food we are eating doesn't have many nutrients to offer, it will actually cause more stress on the body than help the body. The body ends up having to use nutrients it had stored up in order to maintain its daily life functions, and yet it doesn't get anything but a big dose of a highly concentrated ingredient that it will have to work extra hard to process.

Remember that if you want to fix the belly fat problem, eating healthy is one of the *most* important steps. Belly fat is the beginning of the body developing health issues and nutrient deficiencies, we are stopping this process by changing to a healing lifestyle. How can we expect our bodies to heal themselves if we don't provide the tools it needs to do so?

It's been widely known that fried food is unhealthy.

Think about why:

It isn't the food itself that is unhealthy, it's the fact that it is <u>cooked in oil</u>.

The way that oil causes issues is that it frequently contributes to blood vessel and circulation issues.

So what is the connection between our waists and our intake of oil?

Researchers often find out how healthy the functioning of our endothelium is based on the ratio of our waists and hips [92][93].

The thing is, cooking with oil is bad for the endothelium. Even cooking with olive oil has been shown to cause damage to the endothelium, and increase waist-expanding triglycerides [94].

So yes, olive oil may be considered *the best* (for now), but look at the options. When we compare olive oil to walnuts we begin to see that olive oil isn't ideal, but that **whole and unprocessed fat sources** are ideal for our waists and our health [95].

Chicken is thought to be healthy until it's *fried* chicken, potatoes until they're french *fries*, even zucchini is healthy until it's *fried*.

What frequently happens is, when oil is heated, it oxidizes, which gradually changes the oil into trans fats.

Oil itself isn't *totally* bad though, it's the heat, and the act of frying: Virgin coconut oil, when unheated, actually has positive effects on the function of the endothelium [96][97].

It all links back to our actions. If we choose not to fry food, we can make it easier for our bodies to improve from the inside-out which allows our waists to return to a healthier size .

So how can we live without oil?

How can food even taste good without oil?

Here are some cooking methods for cooking without oil:

Always include something that contains a significant amount of fat, like avocados, nuts, and seeds. You can mash them or blend them to make it easy to blend into a dish. Fat helps to disperse flavor in a dish, it really enhances the taste of food regardless of whether it's a healthy fat or an unhealthy fat. When we include healthy fats in our diet, we are helping our bodies to be able to digest carotenoids and other fat-soluble nutrients better, while also satisfying our natural biologically driven need for fat in our diets. To remove oil from your cooking doesn't mean to remove fat from your diet.

Another idea is to make a broth, dressing or sauce and create a soup, salad or stew. Instead of frying food in a pan of oil all the time, cook food in a homemade broth of herbs, spices, water, and salt.

Blend a dressing or a sauce with nuts and seeds instead of oil. Everything doesn't need to be cooked with oil.

Most recipes can be made without oil, all you need to do is make sure to replace oil with something that has fat but is **not highly processed**. It also helps to have a liquid like water or milk to simmer food in.

Another meal idea is to steam or boil veggies instead of frying them. You can add salt and seasonings so that it is still full of flavor. For example, when I make broccoli, I like to steam it and then season it with lemon-herb seasoning. You can even blend up a sauce to drizzle over the broccoli or to dip the broccoli in.

To get a crispy texture in your food, bake it on high heat on a silicon sheet (so that it won't stick). You can use a convection oven/air fryer if you want to get crispness without oil. Your body will thank you for it, by changing from the inside out. For ideas and to get some practice on preparing these meals, make sure to get my recipe book "Belly Fat Recipes and Evidence Based Tips" (on Amazon).

When it comes to belly fat, we have to take a lot of responsibility into our own hands because most food that we find in restaurants and in the grocery stores have ingredients that cause belly fat. Cooking your own food will make fat loss happen so much faster, that's why it's important to have a basic understanding of how to make dishes that are aligned with your health and body goals.

Raw Fats - Balancing the Scales

Now of course there are those who really aren't ready to get rid of fried food, so I'm including one helpful tip. When you eat a meal that includes fried food, be intentional about including *unprocessed healthy fat from nuts/seeds*. Raw fats are good for counteracting negative effects of cooked fats [98].

Eating raw fat from fresh nuts, seeds, and avocados have been proven to prevent and lessen the damage that high-cooked-fat meals cause. Raw fats provide the enzymes necessary to break down the fats into useable components that contribute to the nutrition of the body. Raw fats also promote healthy blood vessels, a healthy heart, and a healthy waist size.

Of course it won't be a perfect fix unless you completely eliminate unhealthy food from your body, but **healthy food makes unhealthy food have less of a negative effect**.

Raw fat (like avocado) helps to prevent belly fat.

This is how: It keeps triglycerides in check, protects blood vessel health, and lessens inflammation.

In this study, just adding an avocado to a hamburger meal prevented some inflammation from happening, kept the triglycerides from increasing, and helped to preserve blood vessel health [99].

Another study showed that 30 grams of mixed nuts eaten daily decreased the participants waist size by 5 cm in one year. *Most people see yearly gains in waist size, but not the nut eaters. They have yearly losses in waist size.* Nuts help to reduce waist-expanding cholesterol and triglycerides [100].

Another study showed that flaxseeds prevent belly fat, lower inflammation in the body (C-reactive protein) and they lower Diabetes A1C levels in the blood. All the factors that flaxseeds reduce are causes of belly fat [101].

Lastly a very large study established that *the more nuts people eat, the less weight they gained each year* (regardless of the fact that nuts are high in calories) [102].

Another study also displayed the amazing health benefits of nuts.

There were 2 groups.

Both were on the healthy mediterranean diet, while 1 group had nuts and the other group had extra virgin olive oil.

Nuts reduced the small bad LDL cholesterol by making them larger, helping to prevent plaque formation, ultimately improving cholesterol. By correcting LDL levels, the waist naturally becomes smaller in size. The nut group as a result, experienced reduced overall LDL levels and experienced a significantly reduced waist size as well [103].

Both groups increased the large good cholesterol HDL levels.

But the olive oil group didn't have the reduction in waist size or LDL level.

So as I mentioned in the introduction, most people gain weight and their waists increase in size every year. One particular study showed that the people who supplemented with flaxseeds for 3 months only gained .6 cm while the placebo group gained 2.1 cm within that time. That's 3.5 times LESS weight gain! So apparently, like the nuts, flaxseeds help to prevent abdominal fat accumulation [104].

Flaxseeds even help to balance out hormones in women by reducing androgen hormones. Women with PCOS and hirsutism (excess body hair) can benefit from supplementing with flaxseeds - about 30 grams a day [105], which can be mixed into a fruit smoothie without affecting the taste in a negative way. Flaxseeds help to make fruit smoothies taste more creamy. Many women with belly fat have excess androgen hormones in their body. So it's important to consider adding flaxseeds to your diet if you are a woman with belly fat.

Lastly, those who eat more nuts gain less weight each year [106]. I must warn you though, that this doesn't apply to just *any* can of nuts. <u>Be careful not to buy the roasted nuts because they add oil and sugar to them.</u> Beware, and check the ingredients lists of roasted and flavored nuts.

Now that we have an understanding of how raw fats and nuts can be beneficial for attaining a healthy waist and preventing weight gain, I want to stress how amazingly effective it is if you make sure to have nuts and avocados <u>every day</u>.

The thing a lot of people don't know about healthy fats, is that they help your body to store fat and lose fat in the *right* places. They aren't actually major contributors to unhealthy weight gain.

Replace Olive Oil with Nuts

For those of you who are still stuck eating things with olive oil, there are some real benefits to be had by replacing olive oil with nuts. People who eat nuts as their dietary source of fat instead of olive oil had smaller waists than those who used olive oil [107]. And as mentioned before, our waists are a reflection of our health. Our bodies just do better with whole forms of food.

Remember, higher LDL levels mean a larger waist.

Nuts protect our bodies by converting the worst forms of LDL (small LDL) into a healthier form, which improves our blood vessel health [108][109]. And if you remember from earlier: higher LDL levels mean a larger waist. So it's quite beneficial to get a regular source of nuts in your diet.

You may also remember that HDL helps to shape the body by lowering the overall waist-to-hip ratio.

Avocados in particular have been shown to elevate this HDL "good" cholesterol which is good for developing larger hips, which contribute to an hourglass shape [110]. A lot of these healthy fats have been proven to correct the way our fat deposits on our bodies.

Tree nuts are also quite significant. They can result in a 20% less chance of having a large waist [111]. That's a significantly reduced risk of developing belly fat. Nuts are an absolutely essential part of our diets.

Tree nuts are also great for satisfying the appetite. Almonds are a perfect snack because they're so filling, and are also known for getting rid of belly fat and lowering bad cholesterol [112]. They're super high in protein which helps you to feel satisfied after eating.

A *daily* dose of nuts is a great habit to put into place. Having just **a handful of raw nuts a day** can be the key to a totally different body, inside and out. Again, be careful not to choose roasted nuts with sugar and/or hydrogenated oils added to them, those can be counterproductive.

Nuts can be mixed into your oatmeal, blended into a salad dressing or a nut butter, or simply eaten plain. Your body will thank you.

*Note: While this may be an obvious statement, please be careful not to eat nuts that you think you may be allergic to.

Different Types of Dairy Products Can Have Different Effects on your Waist.

Many of you may have heard about yogurt being a waist slimming food but it's more complicated than that.

Yogurt *can* reduce waist size - **but** the sugar that is often found in yogurt is a cause of belly fat. If there is enough sugar in your yogurt, you may not get the yogurt benefits at all. It's safest to make your own yogurt or buy plain yogurt and blend in *natural* fruit to sweeten it instead of sugar.

Also, low-fat yogurt does not provide the waist-slimming effects that whole fat yogurt does. Yes, you heard that right, whole fat is more waist-slimming than low fat.

Cheese hasn't been specifically studied that much. Gouda has been shown to improve cholesterol levels, and another study didn't specify what type of cheese it was, but it also improved cholesterol levels as well. The problem is that that same study found that cheese increases C-reactive protein, which is a sign that it causes inflammation, which leads to added belly fat.

So it appears that it may have some nice *short term* benefits, but for *long-term*, beware.

Only Buy Grass-fed or Pasture Raised Dairy

It's also important when purchasing dairy products to only buy grass-fed or pasture raised milk products. Grass-fed dairy products provide a good amount of omega-3 essential fatty acids, whereas normal dairy products have more of the inflammation-causing omega 6 fatty acids that we already have too much of.

In several countries, as a public health rule, milk is pasteurized. The pasteurization process kills bad bacteria from the milk, but it also destroys the natural enzymes that assist with its digestion as well as good bacteria. Without the enzymes, your body is further stressed to have to work harder to process the fats and sugars. A lot of the studies that show benefits to slimming the waist and lowering body fat were studies that involved countries *outside of America*. These other countries have much more widespread use of raw dairy products, unlike America, which uses only pasteurized and ultra-pasteurized dairy products.

So ideally, you should get your healthy fats from avocados, nuts, and seeds, and if from a dairy source, make sure it is whole and grass-fed.

I wasn't sure whether to include information from one study because of the risks associated with high fat dairy, but since I prefer full disclosure and this is about slimming the waist, I thought, "Why should withhold this information?"

According to a 2015 PREDIMED study, "Consumption of whole-fat yogurt was associated with changes in waist circumference and higher probability for reversion of abdominal obesity." [113]

This means that whole fat yogurt is more likely to help with slimming the waist (reversing abdominal obesity) - just remember though, that in the long-term, it may still increase your waist (because it increases the type of inflammation related to belly fat) and it may also still increase your risk of heart failure.

Over the course of an 8 week study, Gouda and Gamalost (specific types of aged cheese) were actually found to help reduce triglycerides and total cholesterol [114].

"the Gouda group with metabolic syndrome had significant reductions in cholesterol at the end of the study compared to the control group, and a significantly higher reduction in triglycerides. The gamalost group also had a significant reduction in cholesterol." [115]

Just to remind everyone and warn everyone, high fat dairy as well as eggs are associated with a greater risk of heart failure [116], so while this waist-slimming information may be quite pleasing to hear, please know that there is *still* health risk associated with these food items. Please be responsible in your consumption of dairy products. I only mentioned the waist slimming results of studies because I'm here to share ways that have been proven to slim the waist. And if you so happen to eat some cheese one day, my only hope is that you will know in the back of your mind that while it may not cause you to gain in the short run, to be careful and limit how much you consume in the long run.

A study done in Luxembourg, Germany found that whole-fat dairy products can slim the waist and prevent obesity [117]. Raw milk is still being sold in Luxembourg, Germany so Americans have to take this information with a little bit of forethought and caution because *our milk is different from their milk*, therefore it may have different results.

You may be wondering by now.. "Since high fat dairy carries the risk of heart disease, will low fat dairy be acceptable?"

In short, no. It's worse:

In an 8 week study, they found that low-fat dairy increases levels of inflammation, specifically, soluble tumor necrosis factor receptors or s-TNFR [118].

This is not a good sign considering that this is another type of inflammation that leads to belly fat, and of course to make it even worse, this particular type of inflammation also leads to tumor growth.

I did a little digging and found that this particular marker of inflammation is found in women who have endometriosis [119]. So it may sound all scientific and unreal, but inflammation is very real and can eventually add up to levels that are found in people with real health problems that cause real suffering. Since dairy products can contribute to this problem, I suggest staying away from them if you want to have a body with the *optimal* level of health.

Before we move on to discuss fats that we *need*, there is a certain type of fat that can be highly detrimental to your health and your waist and needs to be *avoided*:

Trans Fats

If you haven't heard of trans fats by now, this could change your life. Trans fats are also known as hydrogenated oils and these oils contribute greatly to belly fat [120]. You can find trans fats in peanut butter, fried food at restaurants, packaged snack foods, and desserts.

Typical households don't make trans fats when they cook, but when corporations cook with oil, that's when they develop. This is because at restaurants and food companies, they may have hot oil cooking food *all day...* the same pot of oil cooking for hours and even re-used for multiple days. The longer the oil is cooked, the more trans fats develop [121]. Of course this *could* be done at home, however it is less common for people to reuse their cooking oil compared to how much restaurants do. If you do reuse your cooking oil, its very important to stop.

One study analyzed what was causing an increase in waist size over 9 years - and one of those waist expanders was identified to be trans fats [122]. So be careful to check ingredients of food that you eat, to make sure that there are no trans fats, including partially or fully hydrogenated oils.

Trans fats are a big no-no, so now that we've established that, we're going to talk about a type of fat that if you **don't** get enough of it, you can develop belly fat over time. This is something that is so essential that you *need* to include it in your diet or you will face negative health consequences.

Omega 3

Omega 3 is an essential fatty acid that comes from fatty fish and sea algae. And in addition to its many benefits, it has also been shown to help reduce the waist to hip ratio [123] as well as maintain it [124].

Losing weight is supposed to happen a certain way. The belly is supposed to be significantly smaller than the hips, and omega 3 helps with this. It helps the body to put on fat and lose fat in the right proportions and the right places.

If you don't want to lose your curves, but you want to lose mostly belly fat, focus on increasing your omega 3 levels. Women with higher amounts of it helps them to develop curvaceous figures [125][126].

Algae is the best source of omega 3 because it is better processed in the body than fish sources. Fish sources are more likely to grow rancid because processing it isn't as quick as it would be if you were there catching the fish fresh and if you were able to eat it right away [127].

If you prefer to consume fish instead of taking algae oil, make sure to prepare it by baking it and not eating canned or fried fish. This will insure that the Omega 3 fatty acids are preserved. Also don't microwave fish because it will increase the cholesterol content within the fish [128]. The Omega 3 fatty acids in tuna for example, are preserved when cooking and even microwaving (although microwaving it increases the cholesterol); but the omega 3 is lost when it is canned or fried.

Another thing to keep in mind is that a lot of fish oil is rancid or oxidized. Animal studies have been done that show that consuming rancid fish oil can be *harmful*.

Omega 3 from algae oil has no major negative effects except for the fishy after-taste or belch when people take high doses of DHA [129]. The safest overall choice regarding omega 3 supplementation is to make sure to eat sea vegetables like seaweed and to take algae oil supplements (*and* store the supplements in your refrigerator to make sure that they *stay* fresh).

Getting enough omega 3 can be instrumental in helping to protect you from having an unhealthy body fat distribution. It really is important to make sure you are getting enough of the nutrients you've been missing [130].

When people correct their levels of omega 3, they end up with statistically significant results:

According to Cambridge, "Higher plasma levels of omega 3 are associated with a healthier BMI, waist circumference and hip circumference." [131]

Without a nutrient dense diet, it's nearly impossible to have a healthy waist size for the long term.

Chapter Eight

Animal vs plant protein for the waist, what to keep in mind

There are two different types of protein: healthy waist-slimming and the unhealthy waist-expanding proteins.

It's so important to know what types of protein are particularly waist slimming because it will give you power over how fast you can achieve your waist slimming and belly fat burning goals.

Protein is Essential for a Smaller Waist

Protein is essential in order to have a healthy body weight, low body fat percentage, and a smaller waist. Regardless of whether you are plant-based, an omnivore, or anything in between, it's still important to eat enough protein.

There are certain types of protein to beware of: Red and processed meat is associated with weight gain and bad health [132], and seitan/gluten has been shown to decrease fat burning and cause fat to accumulate in mice [133] (whose genetics are overwhelmingly similar to ours), so it's best to avoid these types of protein.

Having more protein in your diet is just as needed as having more whole grains in your diet. Protein helps to make your waist smaller *because* it increases the good HDL cholesterol [134].

Having about **1-1.5 g/kg of body weight per day** is an ideal goal to shoot for.

Increasing protein from 15% of daily calories to 30% cause people to eat less overall calories throughout the day. They end up with less body fat even though they could eat however much they wanted to eat (ad libitum diet) [135].

When people eat a lot of protein, they frequently complain that they become constipated. But there are lots of types of food that have protein that are not constipating: Nuts, which have been shown to be waist slimming, edamame, lentils, peas, and beans, etc.

Beans, in particular, are a really great way to increase your protein because they are full of fiber. People who eat beans have a 23% reduced risk of having a larger waist as well as a 22% reduced risk of becoming obese [136].

Protein is made up of a combination of *amino acids*, what we commonly call the building blocks of life. If you're looking to boost your metabolism then protein is a great way to get your metabolism going faster and stronger.

Animal Protein

Protein is essential for having a healthy waist size, but what types of protein? And who statistically has the smallest waist size: vegans, vegetarians, omnivores, or pescatarians? It turns out that vegans have the smallest waists [137].

Research that was done over the long term identifies meat eating with belly fat. Red meat, poultry, and processed meat cause weight gain, especially in the belly.

Knowing that, remember if you decide that you want to go vegan, make sure to include a regular source of vitamin B12 in your diet or as a supplement.

The more animal products are added into the diet, the higher likelihood of later becoming diagnosed with type II diabetes. The people with diabetes, in order of greatest to least were non-vegetarians, then semi-vegetarians, pesco-vegetarians, lacto-ovo vegetarians, and lastly vegans with the lowest likelihood [138].

So what's the problem with animal protein? Red meat, processed meat, and poultry each contribute to small increases in waist size every year [139]. People who eat a lot of animal protein also have higher rates of death from heart disease [140].

When we compare animal to plant protein, we find that overall, plant protein is better. In fact, people can extend their lifespan and reduce the risk of cardio-vascular death by replacing animal protein with plant protein, especially if you smoke, are a heavy drinker, are overweight/obese, or inactive [141]. Eating plant protein instead of animal protein can help to lengthen your life.

Eating meat has been found to consistently contribute to the risks of having a larger waist, becoming obese, and having central obesity [142].

Men can get away with eating animal protein more than women can, but both sexes are vulnerable to the weight gain effects of eating it. The studies show a weight gain effect with red meat, processed meat, and poultry and not so much from fish and dairy sources[143].

One way in which meat is so bad for our metabolism is shown in how meat consumption leads to diabetes. Meat is a significant source of Persistent Organic Pollutants. Essentially, pollutants accumulate in meat. Our environment is full of pollutants, and when an animal feeds on vegetables with pollutants on them, those pollutants accumulate over the course of the animal's lifetime - just like how *we* accumulate toxins over the course of *our* lifetime. All those pollutants are concentrated in the meat of the animal, and when it gets into our bodies from eating it, the pollutants from the animal then accumulate in *our* bodies.

People who consume Persistent Organic Pollutants are at a higher risk of developing diabetes [144].

According to the World Health Organization "POP's bio-magnify throughout the food chain and bio-accumulate in organisms. The highest concentrations of POPs are found in organisms at the top of the food chain. [145]" Non-vegetarians are twice as likely to develop type II diabetes. And when meat-eaters also have a high fat diet, it seems to result in Type II Diabetes. This association is strong for those who eat a moderate - high intake of animal protein.

Meat endangers lives and sets people up for disease. Choosing to be vegan isn't always about animal rights, sometimes people choose to be vegan for their own wellbeing.

Some people would argue that meat isn't the root problem as to why meat eaters are so unhealthy. The idea is that the true cause of these statistics is because they're observing the effects of the western diet, which is more commonly embraced among meat-eaters. The belief is that the unhealthy items (processed foods and sugary junk foods) within the western diet are what's skewing the statistics.

This study shows that people who eat meat regularly have higher LDL, body weight, and a higher risk of hypertension and higher blood pressure numbers. And even when correcting for the "Western Diet" also known as the standard American diet pattern, eating meat still carries the risk for diabetes [146].

People ages 50-65 who eat a lot of animal protein actually have a 75% higher risk of all-cause mortality, a 5-fold increase in diabetes death and a 4-fold increase in the rate of cancer death. When the protein was from plants, the risk wasn't there, at all [147].

So the question for those who want to continue eating meat is: Is there a type of meat that is healthier than the other kinds (other than fish)? No. But if you decide to have meat, you should have meat that ate *what it was designed to eat.* For example, cows eat grass, they should not be eating grains. The food items that animals eat contributes to the animal's nutritional balance.

Grass-fed beef has more omega 3 fatty acid than grain-fed beef [148]. Grain-fed beef would end up having a fatty acid makeup that is unhealthy for humans, while grass-fed beef would have a fatty acid makeup that is more beneficial to humans.

So now that we've addressed this, let's talk about all the perks of plant protein, and why it's amazing for your health and for the size of your waist.

Plant Protein

As stated earlier, people who eat beans have a 20% reduced risk of belly fat. Unlike animal protein, protein from vegetable sources *lowers* the risk of type II diabetes - research shows that if only 5% of meat calories are replaced by vegetable protein (nuts, beans, etc), the risk of Type II Diabetes is reduced by 23% [149].

● Meat ● Veggies ● Fruit ● Nuts/seeds/beans

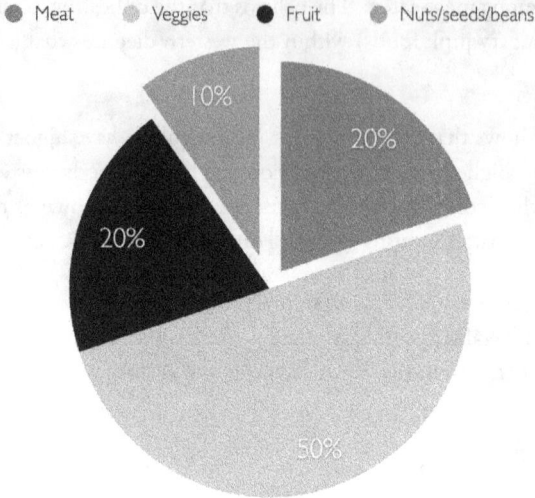

10%

20%

20%

50%

Higher risk of Type II Diabetes

● Meat ● Veggies ● Fruit ● Nuts/seeds/beans

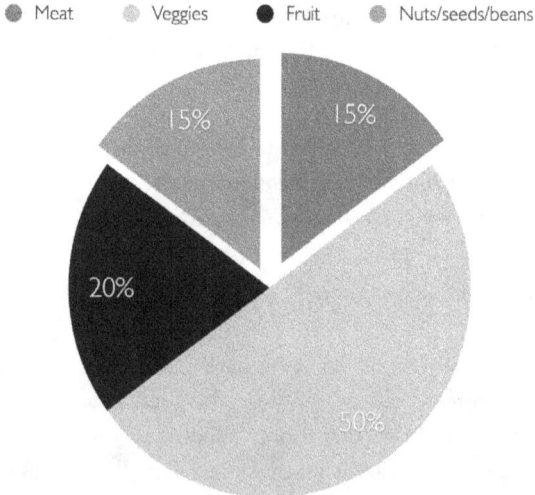

15%

15%

20%

50%

23% reduced risk of Type II Diabetes

Essentially, if we reduce the meat calories to 15% and increase the vegetable protein calories to 15%, we get a 23% reduced risk of Type II Diabetes. If the rest of the meat calories were removed from the diet, that would be a total of 72% reduced risk of Type II Diabetes.

How sneaky is meat, that you can lose weight eating more of it in the short term, but over years and years it can cause you to develop Diabetes?

What if you decided to try eating beans and rice instead of meat?

One study shows the results of weight loss in obese people who eat beans and rice every day:

2 Servings of beans and 4 servings of whole grain rice.

Their waists got slimmer eating this way and they had more nutrients than the control group. The astounding part about it is that their bodyweight was no different between the group that had the beans and rice and the control group. So basically they were able to *specifically* target belly fat while keeping the rest of the weight. [150]

So where should we get most of our protein from? Consider plant sources.

Now you may be thinking, "I can't give up meat altogether", and you don't have to. You can start by eating smaller portions of meat and eating larger portions of vegetables, beans, brown rice and lentils.

When you start changing your diet to be *more* plant-based, you'll see results faster. Remember that even if you replaced 5% of your meat calories with vegetarian sources of protein, you can reduce your risk of developing diabetes, which is related to belly fat. Every little change that you make can have a large impact on the health of your body, and you're in control of what you do every step of the way.

Knowledge is power, the power to determine your own fate and the power to make the decisions that lead to the results that you want. Everything you do can be done *your* way, at a pace that you're comfortable with.

Chapter Nine

Flavoring healthy food with waist-slimming spices

When you commit to living a healthy lifestyle, it's important to come up with a plan that is easy to stick to.

Flavor is something that can't be left out.

Isn't that the whole reason why we eat unhealthy food? Flavor can also be the reason we desire to eat *healthy food*. You don't have to eat plain and boring food, you can make it far more interesting by using spices.

In fact, some spices actually help to enhance the body's ability to burn belly fat.

Experiment with different herbs and spices. Smell them, taste them, mix them in plain food, add a little salt and get familiar with the unique flavor elements they each add to a dish.

I personally find that a good place to start if you don't know how to cook is to simply just use a base of salt, onion and garlic powder. These help build the foundation for flavor in almost any savory dish. From there you can branch out and add other spices and herbs.

Cumin is one spice that is often used in chili bean recipes. Cumin has been shown to reduce cholesterol, triglycerides, *and* LDL, all while increasing healthy HDL levels [151]. Because of that, it has the effect of significantly reducing the waist to hip ratio. When I make a smoothie with a chocolate salted caramel flavor, I only have to mix pitted medjool dates with almond milk, banana, pure cacao powder, and a little salt.

Get to know what specific spices are in your favorite types of dishes, whether it be Thai food, Mexican food, Indian food, Italian or French food.

Healthy food can be made to be just as exciting as unhealthy food. When transitioning from an unhealthy diet to a healthy diet, *remember* your taste buds *will* change. It takes only a few weeks for taste buds to change. Make the transition easier on yourself and get familiar with different herbs and spices.

Let's talk about spicy food for a bit though. Spicy food in particular can be especially useful when lowering body fat levels.

For some reason, spices like cayenne pepper can actually lengthen your lifespan significantly, especially if you're a non-drinker. Cayenne pepper results in a 14% reduced risk mortality when eaten 6-7 days/week. It lowers the risk of cancer, ischemic heart disease, and respiratory diseases [152].

It also reduces belly fat and helps you feel full after meals[153].

It has also been proven to prevent visceral fat from developing in mice, whose DNA is less than 3% different from ours [154].

Spices can enhance the enjoyment of food as well as enhance the body's ability to get rid of belly fat, which improves our overall health and lifespan.

Chapter Ten

Damaging effects of alcohol on the waistline

Damaging effects of alcohol on the waistline

G oing out for dinner and ordering an occasional drink is one thing, but it becomes much more serious when it becomes a *regular* part of life.

Pouring yourself an alcoholic drink on a <u>daily</u> basis could likely be the <u>main</u> reason for your belly fat.

Alcohol *creates apple body types* by increasing the size of the waist, in particular, increasing the waist/hip ratio [155].

Only 1-2 drinks per day, which is also known as "moderate" consumption, has been shown to increase a woman's odds of developing too much belly fat [156].

And when comparing those who drink 28 drinks a week, to those who drank 14 per week, to those who drank 1-6 drinks a week, to those who had none, it is clear that **the more alcohol you drink over the course of 10 years manifests itself on your waist** [157]. It doesn't take very long for 10 years to go by.

Heavy female drinkers, those who consume more than 3 drinks in one day, or those who consume 8 or more per week, are 1.7 times more likely to have too much belly fat for their body mass index (BMI) [158][159].

Heavy male drinkers, men who have 15 or more drinks per week, are 1.4 times more likely to have too much belly fat for their given BMI. As people drink more, their odds of having more belly fat increases [160][161].

Even moderate alcohol consumption is strongly related to belly fat, and obesity in general [162].

If your goal is to lose belly fat, it's important to accept and understand that drinking alcohol reverses waist-slimming progress, and that it increases the risk of heart disease and the amount of fat in the liver - which contributes to metabolic issues and belly fat.

Alcohol doesn't stop there, no. Not only will it make waist circumference measurements wider, it also shrinks the hip circumference because of the loss of gluteal muscle mass and healthy fat stores. Women who had the highest intake of alcohol per week (at least 28 drinks) had smaller hips in proportion to their waist [163].

Researchers now suggest that *the optimal way to drink* is to have small amounts frequently instead of binge drinking. This means to sip at it and not to drink too much or indulge a lot at one time.

The heart seems to handle small, frequent use better than the binging type of alcohol drinking. People with smaller waists and larger hips surprisingly drink more often *but* they just don't drink as much in one sitting. The largest waists were among those who would *binge drink*, and the smallest waists were among those who *didn't drink at all* [164].

If you do continue to drink, consider drinking the alcohol that is paired with nutrition - red wine. And make sure that it is true red wine, because many companies that sell wine add spirits (straight liquor) in there, too.

Real red wine at least has <u>some</u> health benefits from the resveratrol in it, but limit to one drink because your progress will slip away faster than if you don't drink <u>because of the demands alcohol places on the heart and liver</u>.

Wine appears to possibly help improve the waist-to-hip ratio, as long as the person doesn't drink more than 100 grams/day or the equivalent of about half a cup [165]. The people who followed this protocol actually were smaller than non-drinkers and those who drank more than 100 grams/day of wine.

However, remember that alcohol also *destroys* beneficial gut bacteria that are necessary for a healthy body and a healthy metabolism [166].

Beer and spirits are not like wine at all, because there are no benefits, they increase the waist size, causing health issues [167]. Wine has some protective properties in it that counteract the negative effects of the alcohol that's in it.

The benefits of pure wine come from the grape. *Grapes* improve cellular metabolism and reduce the risk of arterial disease [168].

Unlike other types of alcoholic beverages that harden the arteries, wine has a health-promoting effect on the arteries. So if you're going to drink something with alcohol in it, stick to wine.

At this point you may be thinking, "how am I going to do this?" or "this is a lot to sacrifice," but this is about your health more than anything.

Ultimately you have to find a deeper reason to make these changes other than simply wanting to have a smaller waist.

This is about your **health and longevity**.

This is about your quality of life, your energy levels.

This is about having confidence and choosing to love your body by making decisions that don't hurt your life, but that actually improve your life.

The sooner you get started with finding a meaningful reason to make this change, the better off you'll be.

You'll find the motivation to do what's necessary to begin this new, healthier, and happier chapter of your life.

Chapter Eleven

Is salt bad?

P rocessed food is loaded with highly processed salt that is devoid of healthy minerals, but once you've cut out processed food, salt is not a big deal.

When processed food is cut out from your diet, your intake of sodium will *naturally* already be reduced. It isn't essential to quit using salt altogether, but rather to simply quit the salt that comes from processed food.

Salt, with other seasonings, is used to help add flavor and electrolytes to home-cooked meals.

In fact, quitting salt has been proven to be **only mildly effective in lowering blood pressure** because it only lowers it by 2-4 mmHg in people with high blood pressure or heart failure [169].

Salt is an essential source of electrolytes and minerals. You can use Celtic sea salt, French grey salt, Himalayan pink salt, or just plain sea salt. *These* types of salts still have minerals in them.

A meta-analysis in the American Journal of Hypertension concluded, quote:

"End of trial systolic and diastolic BPs were reduced by an average of some 1mmHg in normotensives and by an average of 2–4mmHg in hypertensives and those with heart failure" [170]

2-4 mmHg isn't very much of a difference in blood pressure because it's still *highly likely* that a person can remain hypertensive even after *completely cutting out salt* from their diet.

That's a big sacrifice for a small benefit. There are other more impactful ways to reduce blood pressure (such as cutting sugar intake).

Restricting salt can actually be bad for your health. Reducing it will only lower blood pressure a little bit and yet it increases the risk of mortality in people who have heart failure. Yes, **cutting salt from the diet increases the risk of death for those with heart failure** [171].

So make sure to talk to your doctor about what's right for your specific situation.

Now salt itself, may not be so bad, but there is one type of salty flavored seasoning to beware of: MSG.

Chapter Twelve

The danger of MSG

M SG, also known as monosodium glutamate, is an ingredient that is found in sauces and seasonings such as Accent.

MSG adds a flavor called **umami** - an extremely delicious element to the flavor of food.

So it makes food delicious, but terribly unhealthy.

But just because MSG has umami, doesn't mean that you can't have umami without MSG.

A little salt and natural healthy umami flavors like **mushroom powder**, **tomato powder,** and other seasonings like **miso** (the kind that doesn't have MSG) or **onion and garlic powder** can go a long way in replacing MSG.

People who use MSG are more likely to be overweight or obese and to struggle with overeating because MSG appears to cause something called "Leptin resistance." **Leptin is the satiety hormone**, the hormone that lets our brains know that we are satisfied from our meals. If your body is unable to register when it is satisfied from eating, it will cause you to overeat.

MSG causes weight gain, especially gains in **visceral abdominal fat**. In fact, people who consume MSG are more likely to be overweight, this is *regardless of how many calories they take in or how much they exercise* [172].

MSG has even been found to increase the risk of having metabolic syndrome. One study found that for every 1 gram increase in MSG intake, the risk of having metabolic syndrome and being overweight increased significantly, this is regardless of how much exercise they got or how many calories they ate [173].

That means that no matter how much exercise you get and however much you restrict your calories, you could still be overweight and have metabolic syndrome, simply because you eat MSG.

That makes it all the more important to make sure that MSG isn't a part of your diet, so make sure to **check ingredient labels.**

Chapter Thirteen

The danger of sugar and high fructose corn syrup

C onsuming sugar is another one of the worst things you can do if you want to have an hourglass shape and a healthy heart.

Sugar is literally poison.

It increases inflammation, causes you to store fat in your liver, clots the blood that is supposed to be providing life to your organs, increases cholesterol and triglycerides, ruins heart health, feeds bad bacteria in the gut, and leaves you feeling bloated and tired.

Sugar is sucrose - common table sugar. It has been proven to increase skeletal muscle fat, liver and visceral fat, and triglycerides, which are known to increase the waist size [174][175].

Avoid or minimize sugar at least 95% of the time. It isn't a necessary nutrient, and if you have a sweet craving, you can eat dried fruit or a fruit smoothie instead. Remember that dried fruit may be high in natural sugars but it's full of nutrients and fiber, and it is waist-slimming and health promoting.

If you want to increase the amount of fat that you have, *especially* belly fat, then indulging in sugar is the way to go. But if gaining belly fat is not your goal, leave it alone.

Sucrose isn't the only sweet culprit though, high fructose corn syrup is its evil accomplice:

High fructose corn syrup increases waist-expanding triglycerides, LDL cholesterol, and other types of bad cholesterol, ultimately increasing the risk of cardiovascular death [176][177]. So make sure to avoid this just as much as you would avoid trans fats, msg, and sugar.

Chapter Fourteen

How to read labels

One of the most important life habits to develop in this modern age is reading ingredient labels.

Practicing this habit will help to give you the power to be able to determine what you should buy from the grocery store.

In this chapter you'll practice and learn discernment when it comes to reading labels.

You can take control of your health and refuse to eat foods that rob you of your health.

You'll also be able to feel safer consuming foods that are acceptable to eat. So let's get started.

Sometimes when people look at the nutrition information on the back of food products, they get overwhelmed by the Nutrition Facts label. But the Nutrition Facts label, while helpful, is not the most important thing to pay attention to.

Look at the list of ingredients.

That's where you'll discover the truth of how this food can affect you.

One of the most important things to remember about reading ingredients lists is that the first ingredient listed makes up the majority of what's in the package, while the last ingredient listed is in the smallest quantity.

We're going to go over several ingredients lists to get some practice.

We've already discussed the effects of many types of food, so this is when we put our knowledge into practice.

Some questions to ask yourself while reading labels include:

- Do the ingredients sound like real food?

- Is there anything bad in the list of ingredients to avoid?

- How processed are the ingredients?

Kraft Barbecue Sauce

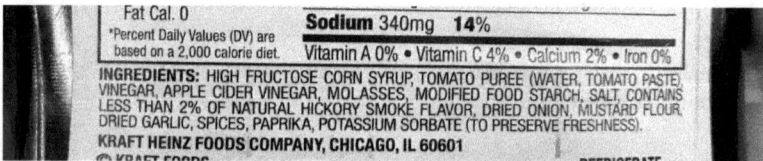

On this label you can see that one of the ingredients that stands out. The very first ingredient is high fructose corn syrup. You know that high fructose corn syrup is an ingredient to avoid.

Another thing you may have noticed is that the ingredients list includes "modified food starch" - which may make you think, "What is that?"

If you ever have to think to yourself, "What is that?" Just know that it is likely something that is processed and therefore is safer to avoid.

Clif Cereal

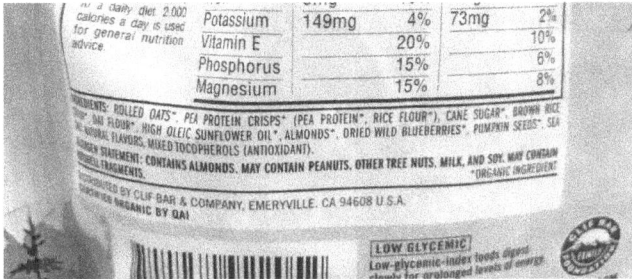

Clif can sometimes be *acceptable* to eat, depending on the ingredients, but it really depends on how much sugar you are allowing yourself to eat each day.

I'd suggest that when it comes to added sugars, limit yourself to no more than 10 grams of sugar per day.

On this ingredients list the ingredients that stand out to me are rice flour (which is likely a simple carb made from white rice), cane sugar (which we know is just plain sugar, which is something that we clearly avoid), brown rice syrup (which sounds processed - syrup should not be associated with food items that aren't really that sweet so it makes you wonder how much processing had to occur), and lastly high oleic sunflower oil (which is an oil: the processed fatty equivalent to sugar).

Crystal Light

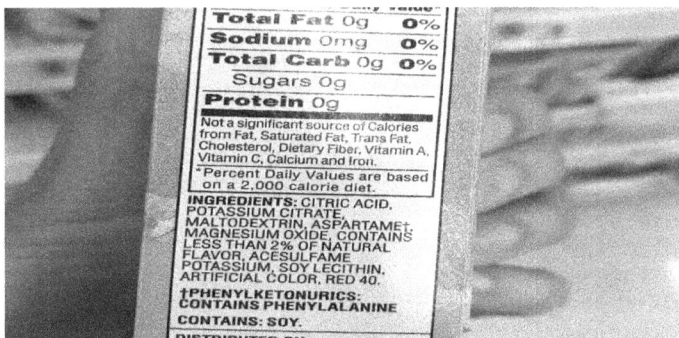

Crystal light is *highly processed*. Just by looking at this label you can tell that no-one can just make this without the assistance of a food scientist or a lab.

It also has unhealthy sweeteners in it like maltodextrin and aspartame, and an artificial color.

Grape Jelly

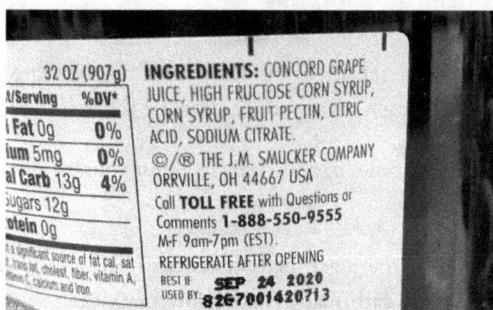

Most people know that grape jelly is going to be loaded with sugar, but a lot of jellies have switched from sugar to its worse counterpart, high fructose corn syrup.

There are also other processed ingredients in it as well. If you're going to have jelly, it's better to have plain sugar than to have high fructose corn syrup. Pick your evils carefully.

Hamburger Helper

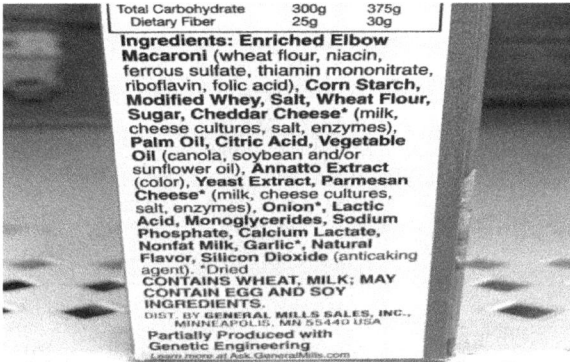

Total Carbohydrate	300g	375g
Dietary Fiber	25g	30g

Ingredients: Enriched Elbow Macaroni (wheat flour, niacin, ferrous sulfate, thiamin mononitrate, riboflavin, folic acid), **Corn Starch, Modified Whey, Salt, Wheat Flour, Sugar, Cheddar Cheese*** (milk, cheese cultures, salt, enzymes), **Palm Oil, Citric Acid, Vegetable Oil** (canola, soybean and/or sunflower oil), **Annatto Extract** (color), **Yeast Extract, Parmesan Cheese*** (milk, cheese cultures, salt, enzymes), **Onion*, Lactic Acid, Monoglycerides, Sodium Phosphate, Calcium Lactate, Nonfat Milk, Garlic*, Natural Flavor, Silicon Dioxide** (anticaking agent). *Dried **CONTAINS WHEAT, MILK; MAY CONTAIN EGG AND SOY INGREDIENTS.** DIST. BY GENERAL MILLS SALES, INC., MINNEAPOLIS, MN 55440 USA **Partially Produced with Genetic Engineering** Learn more at Ask.GeneralMills.com

Many of us decide to get boxed meals because they are super convenient, but you're paying for that convenience with your health.

Boxed items like hamburger helper tend to have a lot of processed ingredients with synthetic vitamins "enriching" them.

You can also tell that it has sugar, cheese, processed milk products, and oils added to it.

This is why it's so important to learn how to season food and prepare it yourself, because you'll naturally avoid a lot of the harmful ingredients in items like this.

A meal like this can be made with pure ingredients at home, and will be significantly less harmful than the boxed version.

Canned Pears

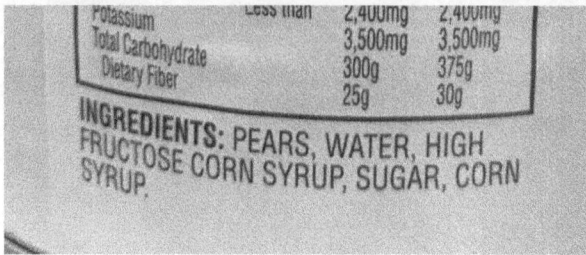

At first glance you may think, "oh these are pears so they must be healthy." This is how people get taken advantage of and conned into damaging their health.

Check ingredients labels *always*.

As you can see, the pears have been soaked in heavy syrup - high fructose corn syrup to be exact, and they even added sugar as if high fructose corn syrup didn't make it bad enough. Look for pears like the ones next.

Healthy Canned Pears

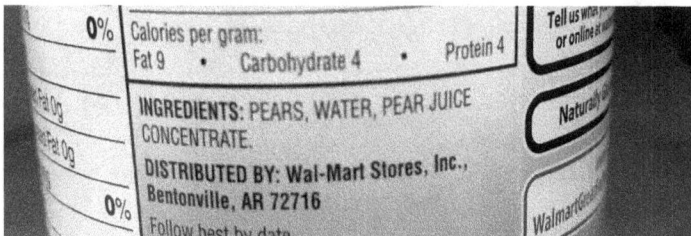

These are the types of canned fruit you would be safest eating. Make sure that they are not soaked in any syrup or sugary mixture.

Make sure they are soaking in pure fruit juice. Natural sugars are what the body is designed to process, not processed sugars.

Okay Ketchup

15	**Cholest.** 0mg	**0%**	**Protein** 0g
0	**Sodium** 160mg	**7%**	

Vitamin A 2% • Vitamin C 2% • Calcium 0% • Iron 0%

INGREDIENTS: TOMATO CONCENTRATE FROM RED RIPE TOMATOES, DISTILLED VINEGAR, CANE SUGAR, SALT, ONION POWDER, SPICE, NATURAL FLAVORING.

This ketchup is acceptable, although it has some sugar in it. Finding a ketchup without sugar and without unnatural sugar substitutes would be ideal.

When you eat ketchup like this (that is sweetened with cane sugar) be careful to check and monitor the amount of grams of sugar in each serving and set a limit of how much of it you will eat.

This one has 4 grams of sugar for every tablespoon of ketchup, so you wouldn't want to eat very much of it: maybe you would limit yourself to 2 tablespoons of ketchup that day. The rest of the ingredients seem fine.

Bad Ketchup

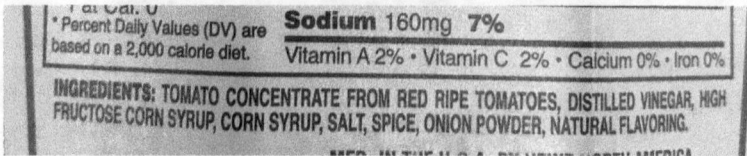

Here's a ketchup that I would advise you to stay away from because it has high fructose corn syrup in it.

It doesn't matter that the amount of sugar is the same, it matters that high fructose corn syrup will cause you to be hungry again much sooner than if you ate a ketchup that didn't have that in it.

High fructose corn syrup has its unique effects that lead to overeating and weight gain. That's why high fructose corn syrup is much more worrisome than sugar (which we also know is bad).

Artificial Sweetener Ketchup

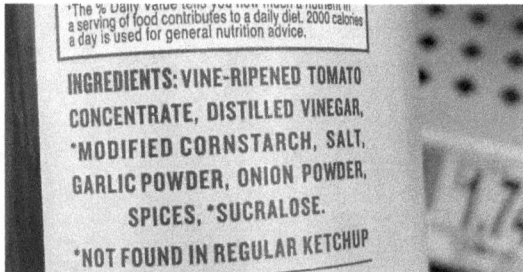

Okay this is the last ketchup I'm going to show you. This one was interesting because it seems very healthy due to the fact that it doesn't have any sugar in it, but most people don't know about sucralose.

Sucralose is worse than sugar when it comes to spiking insulin levels [178] so don't be fooled into thinking this is a healthier option. Also, modified cornstarch is processed.

Sometimes when choosing food options, it helps to imagine that you were a 28 year old who lived on a farm in the 1930's.

Ramen

RAMEN NOODLE INGREDIENTS: ENRICHED WHEAT FLOUR (WHEAT FLOUR, NIACIN, REDUCED IRON, THIAMINE MONONITRATE, RIBOFLAVIN, FOLIC ACID), VEGETABLE OIL (CONTAINS ONE OR MORE OF THE FOLLOWING: CANOLA, COTTONSEED, PALM) PRESERVED BY TBHQ, CONTAINS LESS THAN 1% OF: SALT, SOY SAUCE (WATER, WHEAT, SOYBEANS, SALT), POTASSIUM CARBONATE, SODIUM (MONO, HEXAMETA, AND/OR TRIPOLY) PHOSPHATE, SODIUM CARBONATE, TURMERIC.
SOUP BASE INGREDIENTS: SALT, SUGAR, MONOSODIUM GLUTAMATE, MALTODEXTRIN, CONTAINS LESS THAN 1% OF: SPICES (CELERY SEED), HYDROLYZED CORN, WHEAT AND SOY PROTEIN, TURMERIC, LACTOSE, NATURAL FLAVORS, DEHYDRATED VEGETABLES (CHIVE, GARLIC, ONION), DISODIUM INOSINATE, DISODIUM GUANYLATE, VEGETABLE OIL (PALM), YEAST EXTRACT, POWDERED COOKED CHICKEN.
CONTAINS WHEAT, SOY AND MILK INGREDIENTS.
MANUFACTURED IN A FACILITY THAT ALSO PROCESSES CRUSTACEAN SHELLFISH PRODUCTS.
PARTIALLY PRODUCED WITH GENETIC ENGINEERING.

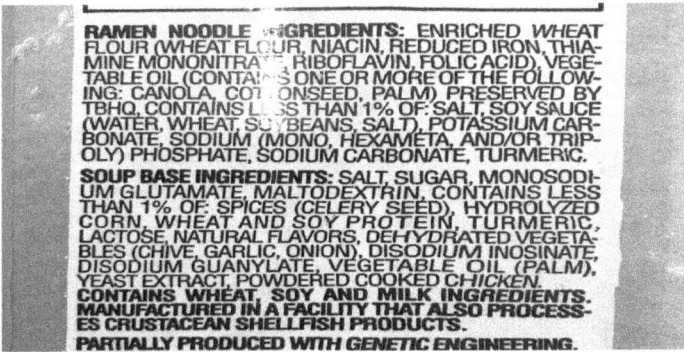

Ramen is thought to be healthy because it's simply noodles with maybe some veggies, but ramen is terrible for the body.

It has highly processed ingredients, vegetable oils, synthetic vitamins, sugar, MSG, and maltodextrin.

Reading the ingredients, it doesn't even sound very much like just noodles and veggies does it? That's how you know it's super processed.

Instant Oatmeal

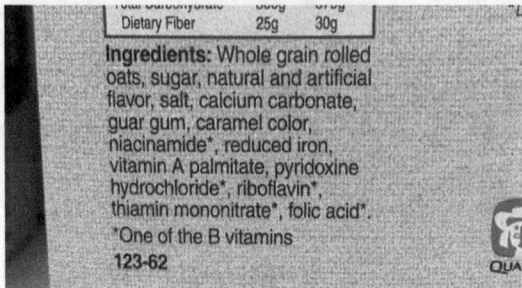

| Dietary Fiber | 25g | 30g |

Ingredients: Whole grain rolled oats, sugar, natural and artificial flavor, salt, calcium carbonate, guar gum, caramel color, niacinamide*, reduced iron, vitamin A palmitate, pyridoxine hydrochloride*, riboflavin*, thiamin mononitrate*, folic acid*.
*One of the B vitamins
123-62

A lot of people think that grabbing a container of oatmeal is okay and healthy, since it's oatmeal after all, but these oatmeal companies frequently find ways to sabotage the benefits of oatmeal.

There's sugar, artificial flavors and colors, and some synthetic vitamins have been added to it.

Folic Acid isn't natural - it is the synthetic version of *folate*.

So please be careful to read labels of food that seem healthy, because those things we overlook are often the main contributors to the downfall of our health.

Peanut Butter

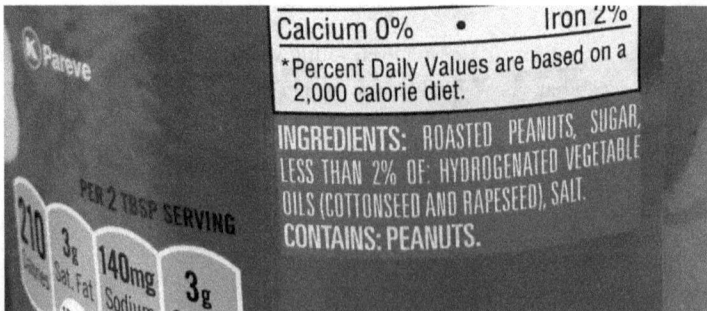

Calcium 0% • Iron 2%
*Percent Daily Values are based on a 2,000 calorie diet.

INGREDIENTS: ROASTED PEANUTS, SUGAR, LESS THAN 2% OF: HYDROGENATED VEGETABLE OILS (COTTONSEED AND RAPESEED), SALT.
CONTAINS: PEANUTS.

Peanut butter is frequently ruined by three common ingredients: sugar, regular oils, and hydrogenated oils.

This particular one has sugar and hydrogenated oils, which are also known as trans fats.

Natural Peanut Butter

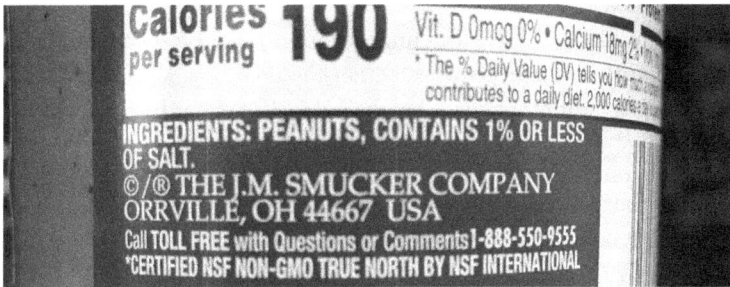

Here's the type of peanut butter that I would advise you to eat instead. It's simply peanuts and salt.

No added oils, minimally processed, with natural ingredients.

Pringles

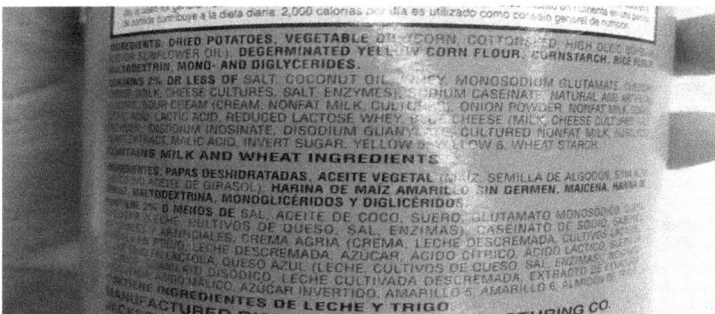

So obviously Pringles aren't the best food to be eating, but I want you to see how bad they are for the body.

They're loaded with simple carbs, they're highly processed, with processed milk products, sugar, artificial color, MSG, and coconut oil has been added to it.

If you want to gain belly fat fast, I'd say grab some Pringles. If not, make sure to leave them alone at least *most* of the time.

During a time in my life I had a Pringles problem. I ate a small can of Pringles maybe between 3-5 times per week. During this time I was walking 4 miles per day and eating healthy otherwise, but those Pringles held me back from making progress.

Take your bad habits and cravings seriously, because they can sometimes be the main thing holding your progress back.

Bad Whole Grain Bread

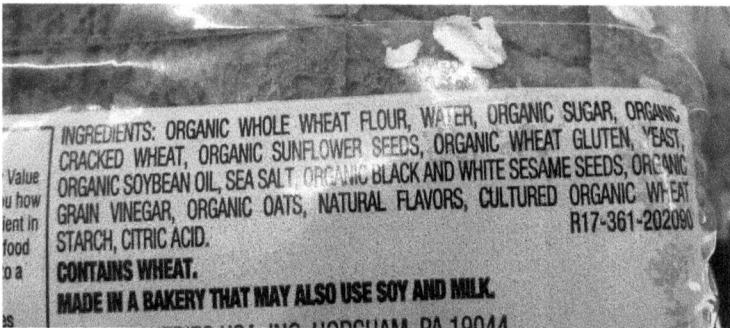

So here's some bread that has healthy labeling and *looks like* it is really healthy. But if you look at the ingredients label, sugar is high on the list, it's the third item on the list, which means they used a lot of sugar in the recipe.

There's also gluten, which, probably due to how processed it is, we know that it can cause belly fat because it slows down the metabolism. And soybean oil has been added to it. Looks healthy, but it isn't without harm.

Good Organic Bread

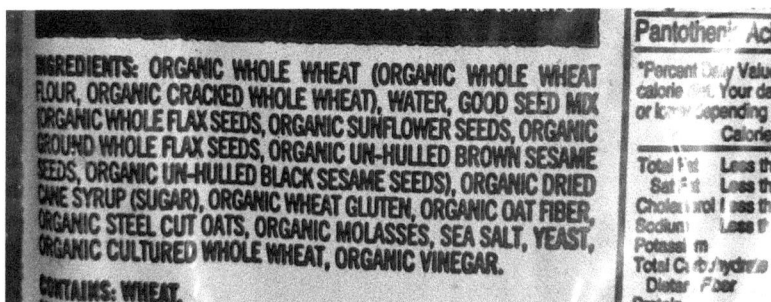

INGREDIENTS: ORGANIC WHOLE WHEAT (ORGANIC WHOLE WHEAT FLOUR, ORGANIC CRACKED WHOLE WHEAT), WATER, GOOD SEED MIX (ORGANIC WHOLE FLAX SEEDS, ORGANIC SUNFLOWER SEEDS, ORGANIC GROUND WHOLE FLAX SEEDS, ORGANIC UN-HULLED BROWN SESAME SEEDS, ORGANIC UN-HULLED BLACK SESAME SEEDS), ORGANIC DRIED CANE SYRUP (SUGAR), ORGANIC WHEAT GLUTEN, ORGANIC OAT FIBER, ORGANIC STEEL CUT OATS, ORGANIC MOLASSES, SEA SALT, YEAST, ORGANIC CULTURED WHOLE WHEAT, ORGANIC VINEGAR. CONTAINS: WHEAT.

Here's a bread that I would find acceptable. For every slice you can see that there are 2 grams of sugar, so if you have 2 slices, you can still stay within a healthy range for the amount of added sugars you eat each day.

Also, the gluten within the ingredients list is lower on the list of ingredients, which means they didn't use a lot of it. The ingredients list isn't *ideal*, but it is probably one of the best breads you will find on the market (in America) due to how natural the ingredients are.

Ideally though, if you're eating grains, they should be whole, like brown rice, barley, millet, and oat groats. That's the safest way because you can eliminate sugar and gluten entirely by leaving the bread alone.

Also when checking labels please remember that *ingredients can change*, so be diligent to continue checking labels even after you have found a good product. Good products often become bad products over time. When products get popular, and the company has to feed more people, they frequently choose to change their ingredients so that they can scale their company.

Now you may be thinking, "There's nothing that's safe to eat!" And maybe there is truth to that. However, we still need to be able to minimize risk so that we can live our lives to the best of our abilities. We'll have to start taking charge over what we eat, to develop cooking skills, and check labels. Do not settle for less for your body.

The sooner you get started with checking labels and taking charge over what you eat, the sooner you will see and feel the results that you're looking for. It really will be a small sacrifice for a great reward.

Chapter Fifteen

Kitchen tips to get started

Start with a kitchen makeover!

Have you ever entered your kitchen and thought "There's nothing to eat" when you know that technically there *is* something to eat? Well that's a problem that can actually influence you to eat the "easy" food which is not always waist slimming. So to prevent this from happening, we do the kitchen makeover:

Get rid of the bad:

Go through your groceries and remove all unhealthy food. Look closely at ingredient labels and remove anything that can cause your waist to expand. Some unhealthy food (only your favorites) can be placed in a separate and significantly smaller section of the kitchen for special occasions or cheat meals. [*Put your unhealthy keepsakes in a small separate section of the kitchen, like a cabinet that nobody ever opens.]

Fill it with the good:

When buying fresh produce, it's best to do the chopping and cutting of vegetables ahead of time. It saves on cooking preparation time and makes it easier to prepare meals quickly. When shopping for healthy groceries, pay attention to labels and if healthy eating is new to you, only choose healthy food items that you like.

The kitchen is supposed to be where healthy eating comes easy! It should NOT be a place of temptation and failure. Food should be well-organized so that you can focus on getting the nutrients you need. When food is well organized, coming up with meal ideas becomes so much easier and saves time.

Also, make sure you have time-saving cooking appliances:

1. Blender - Smoothies, sauces, soups, dips

2. Crockpot & pressure cooker - Cut veggies, add pre-soaked beans and about twice as much water as beans, then allow to cook overnight on low or half a day on high, follow pressure cooker directions, apply salt and seasonings

3. Rice maker - Add rice, water, and seasonings, turn on and come back in about 20 mins. Make sure the bowl where the rice sits is not plastic. Some rice-makers leach BPA into your food, so beware.

4. Nut grinder - Make nut butter or add blended nuts to dishes, sauces, smoothies, or salads.

5. Food Processor - Chop vegetables without effort, make nut butters.

6. Air Fryer/baking rack/convection oven - It's great when cooking without oil, it leaves food crispy on outside. This is not a form of cooking that you should do often. It is a *safer alternative* to pan frying and baking with oil, and deep frying. When food browns, this is called the Maillard reaction. The Maillard reaction degrades amino acids and nutrients in the food. Basically, the more you burn food, the less nutritious it is.

7. Nut/Soymilk Maker - soak beans overnight, blend or strain or place nuts inside with water and wait 20 mins - you can add vanilla extract or use medjool dates to add sweetness. A small pinch of salt can help to balance the flavor.

Your next step in your kitchen makeover will be to stock your cabinet with salt, herbs and spices so that when you're preparing food you are making it flavorful. Some basics that I'd suggest would be salt, garlic powder, onion powder, and cayenne pepper. Also I'd emphasize the importance of having umami such as my personal favorites: miso (without MSG) and mushroom powder.

Remember, this is not a downgrade from your previous lifestyle, this is a proven lifestyle that results in a smaller waistline and more longevity, and it won't be long until you see results.

Seasoning Food is not as Complicated as it Seems

Flavoring and seasoning healthy food is absolutely important to your transition into a new healthy lifestyle because it will help you so that you won't be helpless, having to depend on anyone or anything to continue eating healthy. You'll have the know-how and the basic skills to do what works for you. Because if you didn't have this information, you may have to depend on whatever is available to you. And not everybody knows what you now know.

If cooking is intimidating for you, take a minute and ask yourself these questions. Do you enjoy food? Can you taste different flavors?

If you're like most people, then you probably think this is a silly question because you most likely can (if it's hard for you to eat healthy).

Having that one ability (taste) is the most important element to cooking. If you don't know what tastes good, you can't make something tasty. And if you do know what tastes good to you, then you can make something that you think is tasty.

You may feel like cooking is a very difficult skill to learn but it is essentially as simple as knowing what tastes good and what doesn't. Here are some basic skills that can get anyone in the kitchen preparing food that they like the flavor of.

Salt

This is one of the most important, if not the most important part of cooking. Without salt, flavors get lost and taste very bland and boring. Salt is what brings the flavor out of food. Also for those who are concerned about if they're using "too much" salt: when people season their own food, they don't salt food nearly as much as the amounts found in processed types of food like chips, jerky, hot dogs, crackers, etc. Your overall sodium will decrease from the way you may have been eating before, naturally.

Spices and Herbs

Smell and taste spices and herbs to get to know them better. Our sense of taste and smell are very connected. Typically if you smell something, you can tell whether it's something that is supposed to be used in savory dishes or supposed to be used in sweet dishes. You can tell if it is something you've tasted before or not, and soon it becomes easy when you figure out what spices you like the most. For those who don't know where to begin, remember to try sprinkling a little garlic and onion powder in your savory dishes, then add salt and umami.

Umami

Umami is a flavor profile that engages our entire tongue, unlike other flavors that we taste. It's what rounds out a dish and makes it taste so good you could literally lick the plate clean. Always try to include umami in your dishes. But also beware to avoid MSG (monosodium glutamate) as it is a very unhealthy way to add umami because it increases belly fat. Healthy sources of umami include tomato powder, mushroom powder, umami salt, kombu seaweed, and garlic.

Tartness and sweetness

Adding a little bit of vinegar, tomato, lemon, lime, cilantro or something sweet like tamarind or maple syrup can fix a dish. If you don't know how to fix a savory dish and yet you sense something is wrong with it, try adding something with a tart or sweet flavor. Don't overdo it though, a little goes a long way. Add little by little and taste it each time.

Condiments and salsa

There are times when you'll want to make a quick easy dish or salad. In that case it's fine to buy something that's ready-made, but make sure to read the ingredients label. And remember if it has added sugar in it, to limit yourself to having less than 10 grams of sugar per day.

How long to cook food

Typically when heating food, people cook it until the veggies or beans become softer and the meat is cooked through. You don't have to follow a specific time, just keep an eye on it if you're cooking on the stove and make sure to stir regularly so that nothing sticks to the bottom of the pot.

Once you've developed your first successful recipe, you'll see how capable you really are, and how much closer you are to reaching your goal and having good tasting food while accomplishing it.

Cooking healthy food can be very easy but we sometimes have to give ourselves a chance. When we allow ourselves the chance to cook, we empower ourselves by going through the learning process. Don't let cooking be something that intimidates you from having good health.

You deserve to have good health and to not have to depend on restaurants and junk/prepackaged food.

It's time to taking control over where your health is heading. And learning to cook is one of the most important steps.

Chapter Sixteen

Why you should avoid plastics

I t's important to store food properly in order to have a healthy waist size.

If you choose *not* to store food properly, you will pollute the healthy food that you prepare, and that's not something that you want because it's counterproductive to your goals.

When storing food, always choose glass, especially for food items that are hot or that will need to be reheated. Plastic often contains BPA (bisphenol-A), which causes the body to pack on visceral belly fat, and other types of plastics without BPA haven't been around long enough for us to know whether they're safe to eat. **People with the highest levels of BPA have significantly larger waists** (abdominal obesity, to be exact) **and an increased risk of Type II Diabetes** [179].

BPA isn't just a little chemical to be taken lightly. It's something that we need to seriously avoid. People with the most amount of BPA in their bodies have higher chances of having insulin resistance: 94% higher, to be exact. BPA contributes to obesity, abdominal fat, and insulin resistance [180].

When storing your food, make sure that it has cooled down before storing it in plastic containers. And when reheating your food, move it to a container that does not contain plastic.

While cooking, make sure not to use plastic spoons or straws to stir hot dishes or beverages.

BPA is often found in packaged food, canned food, and food storage containers [181]. It's basically *all over the place.* Maybe you're thinking, "can I even get rid of it?" The answer is that in this society and the way it is structured, you cannot get rid of it entirely, but it can be minimized. Your body is capable of detoxing it within hours to days. But BPA **cannot be completely eliminated** from the body due to unavoidable daily exposure to it [182]. This is still something that you can and should monitor and control for your own health and safety.

Chapter Seventeen

Exercise tips for a healthy waist size and How important is sleep for a healthy waist?

I t's important to discuss how to exercise for a smaller waist so that you don't spend a lot of time and energy doing exercises that really don't result in giving you the shape that you want.

It doesn't matter how much a person weighs, if they're more active, they'll have a smaller waist than someone the same size as them who is inactive. Not only that, but they also tend to have a lower chance of getting coronary heart disease [183]. The size of our waists really do reflect the state of our health. This is true despite variables like family history, age, and unhealthy behaviors like smoking and drinking. And this is true for even petite humans. The amount of physical activity you do matters.

In fact, **the size of our waists predict our death** by disease. In women whose weight is considered normal (BMI between 18.5-25), those with *larger waists* had a higher risk of death than those who were simply overweight or obese [184].

It is so important to be active regardless of what size you are. When people are physically active, they reduce their risk of mortality by a whopping 33% [185].

If you could choose your death, which way would you choose to die? By falling asleep naturally and not waking up, or by some disease that makes you die slowly and miserably?

It's an easy answer.

Our lifespan is something we actually have a large amount of control over, it's just a matter of making choices that benefit our health over those that don't.

Number of deaths for leading causes of death 2017 [186]:

- Heart disease: 647,457

- Cancer: 599,108

- Accidents (unintentional injuries): 169,936

- Chronic lower respiratory diseases: 160,201

- Stroke (cerebrovascular diseases): 146,383

- Alzheimer's disease: 121,404

- Diabetes: 83,564

- Influenza and Pneumonia: 55,672

- Nephritis, nephrotic syndrome and nephrosis: 50,633

- Intentional self-harm (suicide): 47,173

Number of deaths for leading causes of death 2021 [187]

- Heart disease: 695,547

- Cancer: 605,213

- COVID-19: 416,893

- Accidents (unintentional injuries): 224,935

- Stroke (cerebrovascular diseases): 162,890

- Chronic lower respiratory diseases: 142,342

- Alzheimer's disease: 119,399

- Diabetes: 103,294

- Chronic liver disease and cirrhosis: 56,585

- Nephritis, nephrotic syndrome, and nephrosis: 54,358

It is increasingly important to be more active. We aren't supposed to be sitting down all day. Our bodies are supposed to be moving, they're supposed to be actively doing things.

It's almost as though our bodies shut down and begin to die when we are not active.

We have to be doing *something*, we are creatures with bodies after all. What would be the point of having a body if we were not given the responsibility to use it? So we need to use our bodies more often.

Even the small stuff matters. Small, repetitive movements like **fidgeting, can increase a person's lifespan** [188]. Fidgeting helps to increase activity while being in a seated position. So even if all you can do is a little bit here and there, remember that it's helping.

Somebody might be thinking, "my genes are bad though, this stuff runs in my family, there's nothing I can do about it."

Many of us have genetic tendencies that cause us to gain weight in our waists. But that doesn't mean it's hopeless for those of us who do. Research around genetics has improved so much. We've gotten to the point where we're finding out that **our lifestyles influence our genetics**. This is called epigenetics, which means *above* (epi) genetics. So instead of viewing genetics as something unchangeable, consider viewing it as a changeable leaning or a tendency.

Exercise in particular has been proven to be quite effective for people who have genetic tendencies toward having higher BMI's and larger waists. In fact, **those with the strongest genetic tendencies, benefit the most out of exercise** [189].

If you have family with Diabetes, metabolic syndrome, or any other metabolism-related disorder, it's likely that you have a genetic tendency towards metabolic problems. Just know that you aren't powerless. It will take adjusting to a lifestyle that requires you to be a little more active than you currently are, but the rewards are immense.

Cardiovascular exercise is especially important, that includes walking, jogging, skating, biking, and more. Cardio is so important to heart health, and the health of our hearts is reflected on our waists.

According to the International Journal of Obesity, physical inactivity and abdominal obesity were both independently associated with an increased risk of coronary heart disease (CHD) [190]. Coronary heart disease is the narrowing or blockage of the arteries which is caused by the buildup of fatty material. Individuals with large waists are more likely to develop Coronary Heart Disease.

Studies have even shown that very large waists are associated with about twice as high of a risk of dying [191].

Being active helps to reduce the chance of developing heart disease. A systematic review and meta-analysis by the European Journal of Preventive Cardiology analyzed how much of an impact exercise had on deaths of all causes as well as deaths from cardiovascular diseases.

Results from this review showed that physical activity reduced cardiovascular death by 35% and all-cause death by 33% [192].

The recommended time for physical activity for adults between ages 18-64 is 150 minutes of moderate activity, 75 minutes of vigorous activity, or a combination of the two, per week for optimal health [193].

If you can't do that much time each week, remember that even fidgeting can help with lengthening an inactive person's life. With these tiny movements, your body is still able to burn energy.

Even if you don't have time to fit in a good exercise session, fidgeting and every level of activity between inactive and vigorous activity can help!

A simple rhythmic tap, shaking of the leg, or frequent shifting in your seat can actually help tremendously.

Research proves that our waists are a sign of how long our lives will be, and how healthy our hearts are. And we also know that even small movements while sitting lengthens our lifespans. There's something unique about movement and how it's necessary for our health and longevity. We really can't outsmart our body's need for exercise. There are multiple factors that affect the size of our waists and physical activity is a major one. All we have to do is change our mentality to view exercise as a positive and enjoyable activity, and to develop the **habit** of exercising. Make it a lifetime commitment, a commitment to your health, happiness, and self esteem.

Make Cardio a Daily Goal

If there were a pill to get rid of belly fat and improve your overall health, aerobic exercise would be it. It's actually been proven to work a lot like a pill: **the more cardio you do, the less belly fat you have** [194]. Just don't go over 20 miles of cardio per week because that amount has been connected to having a *shorter* lifespan [195]. Choose a cardio plan you can be consistent with, and start with a small daily goal that feels doable before you really push yourself.

Aerobic exercise targets both major types of fat in the belly: the **subcutaneous** fat and the **visceral** fat. The subcutaneous fat is the fat that you can pinch and grab, and the visceral fat is the fat that makes our waistlines look naturally larger because it is the fat that wraps around our organs.

Our natural waists are actually quite small, and typically it's the visceral fat that is the hardest to lose for those who are inactive.

Not only does cardio burn visceral *and* subcutaneous fat, it also burns the fat that is within the liver. Between 10% and 46% of Americans have fatty liver [196][197], which expands the waistline.

And cardio is an excellent way to get the fat out of the liver and to restore the metabolism [198].

Cardio is so effective at slimming the waist that within 8 weeks, participants of one study were able to see their waist-to-hip ratio decrease just by doing cardio in the mornings 6 days per week [199]. That means that just by changing one thing in your lifestyle (adding cardio) you can get more of an hourglass shape.

Another great part is, cardio is something that we can count on, whether that's taking a brisk walk, jogging, or going on a run. What matters the most is the *amount of time* you spend doing it.

For lower intensity activities like walking:

45 mins a day is good.

For medium intensity activities like jogging:

20-30 mins a day is good.

And for high intensity activities like running:

10-20 minutes per day is good [200]. Stick to it and you'll see the results fast.

If cardio seems especially difficult for you, focus on perfecting your diet so that you can prepare yourself and heal beforehand. Exercise can be introduced later if needed, and fat loss can be achieved regardless of whether a person is active or not.

What about HIIT?

High Intensity Interval Training (HIIT) typically involves sprinting, plyometric exercises, and/or resistance exercises done at a fast speed or with little to no time to rest between lifts.

HIIT has been shown to lower insulin resistance and improve glucose tolerance in the body. It destroys body fat and increases your oxygen uptake or V02max [201].

Also, if you're overweight, you may believe that high intensity interval training burns fat extra fast, and yes it does, but for overweight people, it doesn't burn as much BELLY fat as **continuous aerobic exercise** [202]. HIIT may increase the risk of injury. HIIT is better used to save time and to get a quick workout in. But continuous exercise such as a brisk walk is more effective for reducing *belly fat*.

If you've been exercising for awhile and you have a low risk for injury and want to do HIIT, there are lots of benefits.

One study compared:

2 days of HIIT training plus 2 days of regular gym training

to

4 days of regular gym training only

...and while both were effective, the HIIT group improved cardiorespiratory health better and got rid of belly fat faster [203]. So basically it's better to do 2 days of HIIT and 2 days of regular gym training per week than perform 4 days of regular gym training alone.

Gym training is kind of a vague term though, the study didn't say whether gym training includes cardio or not but I doubt it did because gym training is typically used synonymously with resistance/strength training.

Ultimately the most important lesson to take from it is to adopt an exercise routine that is doable, one that you can do consistently and that isn't too hard for you. If you push yourself too hard, you could push yourself out of wanting to exercise at all.

Now, it's super important to build the muscles in our lower body because in this society, it's easy to do too much sitting and not enough movement. To balance out how inactive we are, we need to place extra emphasis on the areas of our body that tend to be less active.

Targeting Glutes During Lunges and Squats

Sometimes when we exercise our legs, we feel the front of our thighs (quads) burning, but we don't feel the actual muscle that needs to be targeted *more*, the muscles we sit on all the time: the glutes and hamstrings (the butt and back of thighs).

The problem is, if you aren't targeting the right muscle, you're not going to see results in that muscle. So that is why it's super important to make sure that you're performing exercises correctly. If you feel as though you're not able to target the right muscle group, it's likely that your technique is off. And if you're really trying to grow your glutes, it's essential to be aware of these 3 things:

1. While performing squats and lunges, **make sure that your back is upright** and not hunched over, it's good to lean forward *a bit*, but make sure your back is straight enough that you look seated upright and a line could be drawn parallel to your back (no rounding/hunching/excessive forward lean).

Don't tilt your pelvis forward or backward, maintain a neutral hip. This helps take some of the work off of your back, preventing back problems and it places more of the load on your legs and glute muscles.

2. Another very important tip is to **shift your body backward**. By keeping your knees behind your toes, your butt will be forced to shift backward so that your body can rebalance itself into the correct position that will stimulate and fire your glutes. It helps to use a mirror to make sure that you are doing this correctly, because if your knees go past your toes, it places the load more-so onto the quads instead of allowing the posterior muscles (hamstrings and glutes) to do most of the work.

3. Lastly, it's important to **make sure that you're actively tuning in to your body sensations as you perform the exercise**. Be aware of where your muscle is contracting and be aware of the positioning of your body and how that affects the muscles that you feel when you move in different ways. Sometimes it helps to actually take your hand and place it on the areas that are contracting to see if they feel hard, then you know that you're activating that muscle. It's all about making yourself familiar with your body and how your movements affect different muscle groups. Forming a mind-body connection is a key element to building strength.

Sometimes we lose touch with our bodies when we don't use them enough, but when we perform the exercises over time, we begin to familiarize ourselves with our bodies again. Once you get the technique right, you'll notice over time that the muscles that you activate regularly will shape up and get stronger.

One very important key to remember when trying to build your glute/leg mass is that you need to do what you can to **prevent your body from feeding on those muscles**. You never want to be in a state of muscle breakdown (catabolism).

Preventing the Loss of Glute/Leg Mass

In order to properly fuel your newly constructed muscles, make sure to get adequate protein and complex carbohydrates to help prevent muscle loss.

Loss of muscle can cause fat levels in the body to increase because muscle is the backbone of the metabolism. Muscle is what burns up most of the calories that we burn everyday.

Prevent muscle loss and weight gain by making sure that you are consistently fueling your body with healthy carbs, protein, fruits and veggies.

Carbohydrates help to prevent the body from burning muscle for energy, so if you cannot get adequate protein, make sure to get adequate carbohydrates from complex carbohydrates like oat groats, brown rice, sweet potatoes, and barley.

Animal protein is great for reaching your protein requirements *easily* but remember that animal protein also causes small increases in waist size over time while also increasing the risk for type II diabetes. Make sure that you are consistently eating a lot of vegetable protein like beans, nuts, and lentils.

People with large waists tend to have a muscle to fat ratio that is off balance. A muscle to fat ratio that is not ideal is associated with [204]:

- larger waist size

- higher blood pressure

- abnormal lipids

- elevated glucose

- and arterial stiffness.

This is why it's so important to maintain your muscles and minimize fat development in the body. And it's totally controllable by your lifestyle.

Carbohydrates are absolutely essential for maintaining muscle mass in the legs because even when protein intake is low, carbohydrates prevent the loss of muscle [205]. Carbs help to prevent the breakdown of muscle because they are the preferred source of energy from the body. Adequate and proper fuel to the body helps to prevent the body from entering a catabolic or breakdown state of being.

Vegetables in general help to preserve muscles. People who eat the least amount of vegetables are at higher risk of having low muscle mass [206]. Protein is still very important for building muscle, but if you want healthy muscles, protein isn't the total answer, it is only an essential part, just like vegetables, fruit, and complex carbs, because without them, the risk of losing muscle increases.

Essentially, if you want to maintain healthy strong muscles over time, make sure you are fueling your body properly and consistently.

Chapter Eighteen

Why you should have an eating bedtime

An important key to having a healthy body with minimal belly fat is to set an eating bedtime. This can be a difficult adjustment, so we will finish this section by going over ways to manage cravings.

It's been known that eating late isn't good for the health, but did you know that it can also cause digestive issues, sleep problems, and weight gain? It's important to eat your meals *way* before you go to sleep.

Eating late can feel like the right thing to do because it satisfies your hunger, but our bodies are not designed to digest food in an efficient way while we sleep. Eating late causes a spike in insulin, even if it's a protein-based snack [207].

Eating at nighttime is also a predictor of future weight gain, even in those who are *not diabetic* [208]. Our health is typically headed towards either a healing direction or headed towards a damaging direction, and if your lifestyle encourages diabetes, one day you may end up with it.

A large amount of weight can be lost just by changing your eating pattern to be **daytime based** and not include nighttime eating. Essentially, we're talking about doing a daily nighttime fast. Eating all your food early in the day is associated with better health and a healthier weight [209].

In one study, women who ate less than 30% of their calories after 5pm had less inflammation (C-reactive protein) and less risk of diabetes (lower HbA1c levels) [210].

Eating late actually shortens the amount of time that you get quality sleep, and it also increases your risk of diabetes. Why is it so beneficial to have an eating bedtime, though?

It's our gut.

Eating right before bedtime causes our gut to have to work throughout the night. **When we stop eating for the night, we allow our gut to rest**. Doing this actually improves gut health by reducing gut permeability, which indirectly helps with obesity [211]. Imagine having to work overtime with no possibility of rest. That's what we do to our stomach and intestines every time we make it work throughout the night, when it's supposed to be getting sleep like the rest of the body.

So what do you do about late-night cravings?

You have to **prevent** the cravings.

Eat a very filling meal around 6pm. - A healthy meal, of course. This works well as a cut-off time for eating. It allows your body to have enough time throughout the night to be able to rest and repair itself so that the body can lose unhealthy weight and remove toxins. If you can't do a 6pm meal with a 10pm bedtime then you can always follow this general rule: No eating within 3 hours of bedtime.

If your body is used to eating late, you will likely become hungry at night, so to prevent this from happening, stay hydrated! This will keep you full and turn off the hunger signals. And by hydrated I mean gulp that water down! Don't just take a sip and then put it back down. By drinking ample amounts of water, your stomach will feel satisfied. The stomach has **stretch receptors** that let our bodies know that we are full and satisfied, so make sure to drink enough water to make yourself feel full/satisfied. This should last for about 45 minutes at a time. It will be difficult at first but with this method, it feels much more doable. Over time, your body will adjust to the new eating bedtime, it can take as little as a week to adjust.

For those of you with stubborn weight, this method can be extremely effective. Notice how well your stomach begins to feel and notice how your sleep improves over time. When you give your gut a rest, your body will repay you.

By now you know that having a healthy waist is a multifaceted lifestyle, and sleep is a very essential part of it. Sleep has a major impact on the size of our waists and our overall health and quality of life.

Sleep is one of the most important factors involved in maintaining our ability to lose body fat. The body does a lot of resetting and restoring during the time in which we're asleep. If the body doesn't get the chance to do this optimally then it will take longer to achieve the same results.

Those who have belly fat tend to get less sleep [212]. The types of sleep that are especially important when it comes to getting rid of belly fat are **slow wave sleep** and **rapid eye movement** [213], this means that it's absolutely important to get *deep sleep*.

Some studies say that the sweet spot to getting *adequate sleep* is to get between 6-8 hours of sleep, however, **7-9 hours per night is ideal for a *healthy waist size*** [214][215].

Commit to getting 7-9 hours of sleep every night. **Sleeping for *less* than 7-9 hours a night can mean that your waist could be *3.4 cm larger* on average than those who get adequate sleep**, assuming the rest of your lifestyle is identical [216].

Our bodies have to *heal* while we sleep, and if we aren't giving our bodies the chance to recharge and renew, then we're endangering our health. Getting enough hours of sleep and enough quality sleep during those hours should be high on your list of priorities.

Here's how to make the change:

- **Set a bedtime**

The body works on a certain amount of energy each day, which is why we get tired around the same time most days. If your goal is to go to bed earlier, set a time that allows enough hours of sleep and a decent wake-up time that fits your schedule.

- **Practice healthy bedtime respect**

Don't get distracted or negotiate with yourself about going to bed later. Set a bed time and stick to it. The last thing you want to do is betray your own trust by ignoring your goals. Your body wants a schedule so that it can get into a routine.

Routines are easier for the body to stick to. Choose a routine and don't make many exceptions. Always return to the routine if you've had to change your sleep hours temporarily.

- **Develop bedtime/relaxation habits**

Minimize background noise - try using a fan to drown out background noise. Sleep in the dark - sometimes the body can't get tired unless it is in the dark, a sleep mask can be helpful if there's too much light in the room. Try drinking herbal tea (without caffeine) before bedtime, avoid TV and other screens for an hour before bedtime, and/or take a bubble bath right before bed to get in the mood to sleep.

- **Wait until the body adjusts**

Lastly, give your body the time that it needs to make your new bedtime feel natural and normal. Just stick to going to bed at the same time even if sleep doesn't come yet and get through the rough adjustment phase. Your body has to get used to it, then it will become your new sense of normal.

- It's also important to note that alcohol and caffeine have effects on your sleep that can shorten the duration of your sleep time and cause you to get lower quality sleep. So make sure to avoid having caffeine after 12pm (or avoid it altogether) and minimize how often you drink alcohol.

Our bodies are capable of adapting to different sleep schedules, but we don't normally give our bodies the chance to adjust. The body has a lot of healing to do when recovering from a belly fat promoting lifestyle. Remember that this is only a phase and that as you continue to stay consistent, your sleep schedule will adjust and you will actually begin falling asleep sooner and getting better quality of sleep than you've ever imagined possible for yourself.

Chapter Nineteen

The impact of smoking on the waist

S moking is widely known to be harmful to our health and to the environment, but did you know it can also rob a person of their hourglass shape? In fact, for every cigarette a person smokes each day, their body weight and waist-to-hip ratio both increase [217]. Cigarettes literally cause belly fat to accumulate in the body.

Current smokers and those who recently quit can attest to it. In a study done with twins, they identified that current smokers and people who recently quit smoking have more belly fat than nonsmokers and former smokers [218].

And that's not the worst of it either. Not only does smoking add belly fat, it shrinks your hips. This technically means that it results in the loss of muscle and and the loss of the healthy gluteofemoral fat.

The size of our hips has a lot to do with our HDL cholesterol levels. And smoking is terrible for that. **Smokers have 1.2X increased odds of having smaller hips than someone else of the same weight/height category** [219]. So basically what happens is when people smoke, they gain belly fat and their hips shrink at the same time. This is the development of an apple-shaped figure.

Quitting smoking can help to allow the body to return its HDL levels by increasing them [220], which can help return your hip size to normal and reduce your risk of cardiovascular disease [221]. Quitting can also improve endothelial function (the inner lining of the blood vessels), which is good for a healthy waist size. So the negative effects of smoking don't have to stay forever.

If you smoke and don't feel confident and capable of quitting, seek support. Consider joining a smoking cessation program. There are too many benefits to be had from quitting.

Now some of you may be thinking that I'm only referring to the effects of tobacco, but there's also research that shows that smoking **cannabis** can result in the development of visceral belly fat, too. Chronic smokers of cannabis also tend to eat more processed carbohydrates, probably due to giving into the cravings of the notorious "munchies."

They also have lower HDL healthy cholesterol levels, which means smaller hips, **any type of smoking is bad for the waist,** and it's likely that you simply shouldn't put any type of smoke in your lungs [222].

We already know that **higher VO2max** levels, which is oxygen uptake, **leads to smaller waists**, so putting smoke in our lungs is not going to help with that. Just to be safe, decide to quit smoking, or do it far less often.

Chapter Twenty

Herbs, vitamins, and supplements for a healthy waist & insights on the gut microbiome

I n this lesson we're going to be talking about herbs, vitamins, and supplements that have been proven to help get rid of belly fat as well as touching on how to resolve belly fat by looking at gut health. This knowledge can empower you to speed up the process of losing belly fat with less effort.

Vitamin D3

Vitamin D deficiency has become something of an epidemic. The majority of the sunlight hours are spent indoors at work, so most of us don't get a chance to just relax and soak up the sun. Naturally, as a result of this, we have a lot of people who are deficient in vitamin D.

The body makes vitamin D in the liver after exposure to the sun.

Without enough Vitamin D, the body develops issues with glucose metabolism, rising levels of triglycerides, non-alcoholic fatty liver disease, the waist expands and the body loses muscle [223][224][225]. All of these issues develop over time as Vitamin D levels decrease. But as levels are corrected, these issues slowly resolve.

Some people may have difficulty correcting their levels of vitamin D because liver health is an important prerequisite to vitamin D. Your liver health could be sub-optimal, like so many of us who go undiagnosed with fatty liver disease from consuming too much sugar, refined grains, and alcohol [226].

Check with your doctor to **see if you may be deficient or insufficient in vitamin D**, and make sure that your liver health is in good order. It's important to fit some time in your daily schedule to allow the sun to contact your skin by taking in the sun rays or by supplementation.

When Vitamin D levels are ideal (50 ng.ML - Nanograms per milliliter), people experience peak athletic performance, their fast twitch muscle fibers increase, and the elderly have less likelihood of falling [227]. It's important to know that this vitamin cannot be created without a healthy liver. Avoid sugar, alcohol, unhealthy fatty foods, refined grains, and make sure to consume sea vegetables to enhance your liver's ability to make vitamin D. This vitamin is so essential to our health. Make sure to get your levels checked and monitor how much sun you get more diligently.

So the question is, can you supplement with it if you can't get full-sun exposure as regularly as your body needs?

Yes. In fact, **supplementation with Vitamin D increases exercise performance and reduces the waist-to-hip ratio**, resulting in more of an hourglass body shape [228].

One study tested the effectiveness of Vitamin D supplements for their ability to improve issues within the metabolism. They found that Vitamin D improved the body by decreasing the participants' waist size, body weight, systolic blood pressure, BMI, and their level of insulin resistance.

They concluded that **Vitamin D2 at 20,000 iu** or **vitamin D3 at 15,000 weekly** helps to improve the body shape of pre-diabetic people [229]. Pre-diabetics are people who have elevated glucose levels - and it's easy to have elevated glucose levels (you can think you're living a healthy lifestyle and still be pre-diabetic). If you are not sure which one to take, **D3 has stronger waist slimming effects** [230].

Rosehip Extract

Rosehip extract may be a little more difficult to find, but for those who can get their hands on it (or even make it themselves) it's been shown to be quite effective at getting rid of abdominal fat, both visceral and subcutaneous fat. The participants of the study took 100 mg/day and ended up with significantly less abdominal fat at the end of the 12 week study, compared to the placebo group [231].

Rosehip is actually a plant with a large amount of Vitamin C in it. This may be the or at least one reasons why the study participants lost so much belly fat, since Vitamin C has already been shown to be helpful for losing belly fat.

Seaweed

Seaweed is so important because it contains multiple waist-slimming and health-promoting components: carotenoids like fucoxanthin, a significant source of natural iodine, EPA, fiber and other anti-obesity components [232].

Most Americans have *subclinical* iodine deficiency [233]:

- people who have **metabolic issues**,

- people who are **overweight**, and

- people with **belly fat**

These are the people who tend to be lacking sufficient iodine in their bodies and in their diets.

It has been shown that supplementing with seaweed helps correct iodine levels [234]. **Increasing intake of seaweed results in a smaller waist** [235]. I would suggest getting iodine from seaweed rather than supplements because seaweed is a natural source of iodine and our bodies are built to process natural sources of nutrients. Seaweed also makes a great alternative to salt and a great complement to salt that does not have iodine added to it such as Himalayan or Celtic sea salt.

Seaweed is especially helpful for women who have estrogen dominance because the iodine helps to lower estrogen to normal levels. There is a strong inverse relationship between seaweed and the hormone estradiol. This means that when people consume high amounts of seaweed, there are low amounts of estradiol, and that when they consume low amounts of seaweed, there are high amounts of estradiol. The study that determined this found that the proper dose was 75 mg per kg of bodyweight. This is between the suggested range to prevent breast cancer. (5-7 grams/day) [236].

It could be the iodine in seaweed that is making the difference with hormones and cancer prevention. When people isolate iodine instead of just supplementing with seaweed, they find that there are also strong anti-estrogen effects as well [237].

Fucoxanthin is a marine carotenoid found in brown seaweed - Supplementing your diet with *this* significantly reduces body weight, visceral fat, and BMI. They compared the placebo, the 1 mg, and the 3 mg, and found it most effective at 3 mg a day [238].

Metabolic syndrome is less common in some Asian countries that consume a lot of seaweed.

One study tested to see how much of an effect supplementing with seaweed has on the waist: In 1 month the participants blood pressure decreased 10 mmHG when they took 6g of seaweed per day. Women's waists decreased by 2.1 cm when they took only 4g/day of seaweed. When they took 6g/day their waists decreased by a total of 3.9 cm [239].

It may be that Seaweed is so effective because of it's health-enhancing effects on the thyroid. When people are deficient in iodine, they develop thyroid nodules, and sea vegetables are a fantastic way to prevent thyroid nodules due to its rich source of iodine. A lot of people with metabolic syndrome or those who have large waist measurements or high triglycerides have thyroid nodules (so it's likely that in order to have a healthy metabolism, we need to eat sea vegetables)[240].

Even people with *normal* functioning thyroids have higher levels of TSH and free triiodothyronine (Try-Ay-Uh-Doe-Thy-ruh-neen) — which is an indication of a need for iodine.

Essentially, larger waists, bad health and body fat are ways that our bodies give off signs that we need iodine [241].

Maca

Maca is a really popular supplement among women who want to develop more of an hourglass shaped body. There's a lot of anecdotal evidence for maca (Youtubers talking about how it transformed their body so that they had slimmer waists and bigger butts) but there isn't much research on it, there is one study, that suggests that there may be some truth to the effects that people say maca has on their bodies.

In this study rats were given Maca, and the effects of it were that it lowered body weight and triglycerides [242]. And we already know that triglycerides influence the size of the waist, and that rats have close genetics to humans. Considering these impacts, it may be worth trying.

Xanthigen

I'm not sponsored by Xanthigen but I did do research on it because it's only a mixture of brown seaweed and pomegranate seed oil, which you can get separately if you wish. It's been shown to slim the waist in people who have fatty liver, it improves liver function, reduces a person's total body fat percentage, and increases the healthy fat-burning brown fat resulting in an increase in total resting energy expenditure [243][244].

It's more effective in people who don't have the clinical diagnosis of fatty liver, because their livers are healthy enough to be enhanced faster. But fatty liver is extremely common, affecting a significant chunk of the US population, and many of us who have fatty liver have *no symptoms.*

Yacon Syrup

This is one that tastes really good (like brown sugar) and it works well as a sugar substitute. It's comes from the root of a perennial daisy that is found in South America. It helps with regularity because it is a good source of pre-biotics which help to make the waist smaller [245]. Make sure to get it from a reliable source as some companies sneak other ingredients in because most people don't know what it tastes like.

So not only is yacon syrup *not harmful*, but it's **sweet** enough to use as a sugar substitute. Yacon syrup has been shown to significantly decrease body weight, waist size, and BMI. It also increases defecation frequency and the feeling of being full after eating [246].

Katemfe, also known as Thaumatin Extract

This may also be hard to find, but it can be found in some health food and supplement stores. Katemfe fruit is found in the rainforests of West Africa, and the protein extract is about 100,000 times sweeter than sucrose on a molar basis [247]. One drop is enough to sweeten a cup or two and it's also non-toxic, so it is safe to eat.

Black Tea/ Pu-er

Before explaining the waist-slimming benefits of black tea, it's important that I remind you that black tea has caffeine in it, limit yourself to no more than 1 cup a day (in the morning before noon), in order to get a good restorative night's rest.

In reference to the study, the participants consumed more than one serving a day. For eight weeks, participants consumed 3 servings of black tea daily. At the end of the 12 weeks they lost visceral belly fat and also lost weight overall [248].

This study on black tea found that black tea helps prevent metabolic syndrome by lowering blood sugar, lipids, and belly fat. Even markers of inflammation were lowered when people took black tea [249].

Remember, if you go to a restaurant and order some type of drink with black tea, it may be **loaded with sugar**. So as usual, in order to keep it healthy, you can make your own or just have it plain. Otherwise, if sugar is in it, it is considered a cheat meal.

While there are benefits to supplementing with black tea, it's important to give your body a chance to have rest from caffeine. Caffeine can be quite harmful to heart health, so in the short term someone may lose weight, however, they may gain it all back in the long run by sabotaging their heart health with caffeine. So make sure to watch how much caffeine you consume.

Seabuckthorn and Bilberry

If you can get your hands on these berries, you can try these out for their waist slimming effects. Sea buckthorn is especially interesting because while the participants were taking these berries, they ate more sugar and fatty foods and **still saw their waist size decrease**. Sea buckthorn is very sour and **full of Vitamin C**, which is a waist slimming vitamin.

Bilberries are another waist slimming fruit which are similar to blueberries but are grown in European and Asian countries.

This short study lasted between 33 and 35 days. The participants took **100 grams a day** or the equivalent of 2 capsules of the extract. Bilberries decreased the waist the most: by 1.2 cm within 35 days while Sea buckthorn decreased the waist by 1.1 cm [250].

Goji

Goji berries are another fruit that has been found to be waist slimming. The study didn't specify whether the berries were dried and rehydrated or fresh, but these participants did a 14 day trial of around 4 fluid ounces or 120 ml of a Goji drink called GoChi, and the participants lost around **5.5 cm** from their waists [251]. The results may have been so extreme due to the high vitamin C content in goji berries. **Vitamin C from fruit and vegetables is a potent waist-slimmer.**

It increased post-prandial energy expenditure in a dose-dependent way (which means that it increased their metabolism after eating) [252]. So typically when you eat unhealthy food, your metabolism may slow down- making you feel tired, but this had the opposite effect.

Green Tea

Green tea isn't just a fad, it's been scientifically proven as well, and drinking green tea is a popular method to lose weight and/or prevent weight gain. One study compared two groups of overweight people over the course of 90 days. One group had 2 servings of a regular drink with added catechins (30 mg) and caffeine in it daily, and the other group had 2 servings of high catechin (886 mg) green tea daily (which also has caffeine in it naturally) [253].

Both groups lost at least 5.6 cm off of their waists, and the **high catechin** green tea group lost about **1.9 cm more** than the regular drink group with catechins added. No exercise or other dietary changes; just drinking green tea resulted in these changes. This is significant because although most people gain from month to month, these people had measurable losses in weight within the study.

The difference between the two groups is that the regular drink had 30 mg of catechins, while the green tea group had 886 mg of catechins. So it was really the amount of catechins that helped to slim the waist and get rid of abdominal fat in the participants.

Saw Palmetto

Saw palmetto is a supplement that works mainly for people who have too much DiHydroTestosterone (women with PCOS or hirsutism, and men who are balding tend to have too much DHT - but check with your doctor to see if this is right for you before deciding to take it.)

The way saw palmetto works is that it inhibits the production of DHT [254]. **DHT is the strongest androgen, so inhibiting its production can help to allow fat to finally store in the lower body where it belongs in a woman.**

Hormones play a big part in losing belly fat. Women with belly fat tend to have higher levels of androgens (commonly thought of as male hormones). Androgens are normal in the female body, but sometimes when hormones get imbalanced, the androgens get too high.

Saw palmetto is a 5-alpha reductase inhibitor, which means it indirectly lowers the production of DHT [255].

DHT is an estrogen antagonist or enemy, it fights the DNA expression of estrogen and because it is the strongest binding androgen, it doesn't get removed easily. So for women with excess androgens, specifically DHT, saw palmetto helps to provide balance. Saw palmetto can be helpful for people who have belly fat, hair loss, unwanted facial hair, or PCOS.

When you stop taking saw palmetto, make sure your diet is right because your hormones will likely become unbalanced again without that proper nutrition.

A diet that is high in unhealthy carbs, fats or high in added sugar or alcohol can cause hormonal problems because the body produces DHT **to protect the liver**, and lots of **fat and sugar damage the liver**.

Essentially the body is only trying to protect itself, even if it means that your hormones have to be unbalanced.

Women with excess belly fat commonly have female reproductive system health concerns. Women with PCOS in particular, have a higher ratio of total testosterone to DHT [256].

Metabolic syndrome, impaired glucose tolerance, insulin resistance, and obesity are all related to PCOS. This hormonal imbalance may be why there's more of an android or apple body shape that's seen in people who have PCOS.

While saw palmetto is not deeply studied, it shows potential in its ability to balance hormones, which may result in belly fat loss.

Women with hirsutism and PCOS have higher amounts of testosterone compared to women with normal hormone levels [257]. To be specific, they have too much androstenedione and dihydrotestosterone (DHT). Tumors found on the ovaries or the adrenal glands can cause the body to develop too much testosterone and even a tumor on the pituitary gland can indirectly cause the development of too much testosterone.

Remember how we discussed that dairy causes increases in s-tnfr (soluble tumor necrosis factor receptors)? That increases the chance of developing tumors and ultimately disrupts hormones. **Elevated levels of soluble-tumor necrosis factor receptors are seen in malignancy, autoimmune diseases and infections** [258]. Let this serve as an additional reason why it's best to minimize dairy consumption.

Berberine

Berberine is an antimicrobial, anti-tumor, immune enhancing, glucose lowering and cholesterol lowering spice. It improves endothelial health and it decreases LDL and triglycerides which we know are often the culprits of belly fat. Berberine has been shown to reduce the waist size in those who have metabolic syndrome and it boosts HDL levels, helping to bring the body back into balance [259].

Berberine has been studied for its effectiveness with weight loss. What's interesting about berberine is that it reduces waist size significantly, but does *not* reduce total body weight significantly. There is a dose-response relationship with berberine, it appears that it significantly reduces the waist circumference and body mass index [260].

Neem

Throughout history in India and southeast Asia, neem has been used to fight bacterial, fungal, and viral infections. Neem extracts have been shown to be effective against many types of bacteria, including obesity-associated bacteria like streptoccoccus. Not only is neem a powerful antibacterial, it is also a powerful antifungal. It inhibits the growth of several different types of human pathogens, including Aspergillus and Candida [261].

Neem extracts have also been used to keep parasite eggs from hatching, disrupt their hormones and their ability to eat and reproduce [262][263].

Depending on what type of pathogen may be contributing to belly fat, neem can be potentially helpful.

Things to consider when supplementing:

Obesity with inflammation often indicates an altered gut microbiome. Obesity is associated with less diversity of bacteria in the gut, as well as increased or decreased concentrations of particular types of bacteria and microbes within the intestines [264].

Obese people tend to have larger amounts of an inflammation-promoting type of bacteria called Proteobacteria. Some of the proteobacteria that were identified to increase BMI are E. aerogenes, K. pneumoniea, Vibrio, and Yersina bacterial species.

Among other types of bacteria, firmicutes are more abundant and bacteroidetes are less abundant by threefold within the intestines of obese people. So there are fundamental differences between a healthy gut and a gut that struggles with weight gain. These differences in gut flora may actually explain why obesity is associated with higher levels of inflammation. Research[265] has shown that when obese people have low levels of bacteroidetes, they often have high levels of C-reactive protein which indicates presence of inflammation. Inflammation is not just an invisible force that negatively affects the body. Inflammation happens as a consequence of an imbalanced gut flora.

Another bacterial species called allistipes is far *less* abundant than what is found in the normal gut flora, by over 6 times [266]. Now this doesn't mean that obese people need to start increasing their allistipes bacterial concentration and keep doing so for the rest of their lives, no. Bacterial balance is about balance. Too much of allistipes can be detrimental to health, while too little can also be detrimental to health. It's important to understand that health is a spectrum that we fall into, and that each person has a uniquely different gut flora that presents unique challenges when following a healing protocol.

It's important to be aware that our gut flora has major impacts on our body fat composition and our overall health. Taking your gut health into consideration should help provide the advantage of being able to *solve* the weight issue. If a person follows conventional weight loss advice, but does not take action to correct their gut flora, then they will likely fail in their efforts. For example, if you follow a low calorie protocol that still includes foods that disrupt your gut flora, you will be less likely to see the progress that you're looking for. This is about fixing the root of the problem. If you struggle to lose belly fat then your next step will be to do gut microbiome testing or simply to cut out foods that are food to bad bacteria. Fasting and eating whole unprocessed fresh food can also be helpful for shifting intestinal bacterial balance for the better.

When shifting your gut balance to something that is less obesogenic, it's important to consider consuming a diet that helps to alter the bacteroidete/firmicute ratio. One thing you can do to correct this is to watch what type of fats you eat predominantly. High fat diets can be allowed for a healthy gut flora, but they need to be comprised of less omega 6 fatty acids and less long chain fatty acids to minimize the risk of disease and worsened gut health [267]. If you want to increase your beneficial microbes, make sure to prioritize consuming sufficient omega 3 fatty acids in the form of EPA and DHA everyday.

Obesity tends to result in certain gut changes. These types of bacteria are significantly more abundant among obese people [268]: Acidaminococcus, Anaerococcus, Catenibacterium, Dialister, Dorea, Escherichia-Shigella, Eubacterium, Fusobacterium, Megasphera, Prevotella, Roseburia, Streptococcus, and Sutterella.

As for the bacteria that are not abundant enough: Bifidobacterium, Eggerthella, Bacteroides and Collinsella.

Research isn't entirely clear on how bacteria affects people. Some studies conflict with other studies so we haven't been able to determine whether the following bacteria are obesity-related or not. It could be that the interaction of the different bacteria with one another is what affects our metabolism. So even though results are not clear, it is helpful to take note of what bacteria these are. The bacteria with controversial results are: Akkermansia, Alistipes, Anaerotruncus, Bacteroides, Blautia, Clostridium, Coproccocus, Desulfovibrio, Faecalibacterium, Oscillibacter, Oscillospira, Parabacteroides, and Ruminoccocus.

Fungi also play a role in obesity. Penicillium and Rhodotorula were found more often in overweight and obese people. In general, obesity usually means a higher yeast count. People of normal weight have more gut diversity and an abundance of a type of yeast called Trichosporon [269].

Mulberry leaves can potentially be a helpful herb to take in the form of a tea. Mulberry leaves reduce proteobacteria concentrations and help to correct the ratio of bacteroidete/firmicute ratio. They've been proven in mice to cause fat loss, reduce blood sugar, improve insulin sensitivity, and improve liver and kidney health [270].

Activated Charcoal

Often used to save lives in the hospital from accidental poisonings and used in water filters to purify our drinking water [271], activated charcoal is a tasteless black powder that adsorbs many different types of substances, including toxins that it can deactivate and carry out the body through bowel movements. Charcoal is typically a burnt organic plant material, like wood, coconut or eucalyptus that is burned at extremely high temperatures (400 Celsius/ 750 Fahrenheit) in a pot or container keeping oxygen out [272].

The charcoal that is often found to be the most beneficial is the acidic activated charcoal. This means that after the charcoal is burnt, it is rinsed with an acidic liquid such as vinegar or the juice of fresh squeezed lemons. The result of this process makes charcoal have so many holes in it that attracts or causes microscopic substances to adhere to it. This means that it can get rid of a lot of different things, in fact, this type of charcoal has been found to adsorb heavy metals [273], toxins, and due to its ability to adsorb lipids, it can even disrupt the body's absorption of dietary fat [274]. Of course this cannot be abused, because dietary fat is a necessary part of what our bodies require in order to process our fat-soluble vitamins. But it can be used tactfully in order to lessen the negative effects of certain cheat meals, high fat meals like French fries and funnel cake, or anything else that may increase cholesterol.

It appears that charcoal may also inhibit the development of visceral fat because of its ability to escort fatty acids out of the body [275]. Activated charcoal has actually been shown to have a dose-response effect on cholesterol levels (decreased LDL) when taken between 4 and 32 grams per day [276].

Of course activated charcoal is known for helping with bloating and gas. But it is also known to enhance kidney health, especially among those with chronic kidney disease. It lessens the work that the kidneys have to do by reducing the waste products that the kidneys would have to filter [277].

It also helps in the case of infection; charcoal has been found able to adsorb certain types of E. coli as well as verotoxin [278] and the crazy part is that charcoal is less effective at binding to the healthy and normal type of bacteria that we need to hold onto. How amazing is it that charcoal just so happens to be beneficial in the way that we humans need it to be?

CARDAMOM

Cardamom is a commonly used Indian spice that also has a lot of health benefits.

When studied on rats separated into two groups, it was found that if the diet was the same for both groups (a fat-gaining diet), that the cardamom powder group developed less abdominal fat and less inflammation in their livers than the group that didn't have cardamom powder [279].

In humans, cardamom has been shown to reduce the types of inflammation that are related to having belly fat, including Interleukin-6 and C-reactive protein [280].

Green cardamom in particular has been shown to balance hormones in obese women who had pcos. It helped to lower their androgen hormones, including the powerful hormone DHT and follicle stimulating hormone, resulting in a more normalized state of health. It also lowered markers of inflammation that are related to belly fat: TNF-α, IL-6, and CRP. The most mind-blowing part of it all is that not only did it do all this, but it even changed the DNA expression of TNF-a and CRP [281].

GINGER

Ginger is a root vegetable that can be taken in powder form, as a tea, cooked within food or eaten raw. It has a strong spicy flavor with a penetrating scent. Ginger helps to get rid of waist-expanding triglycerides, lowers the amount of glucose in the blood, increases HDL and improves insulin resistance. All these health benefits to the organs in the body result in outer physical changes. Supplementation with ginger results in a reduced waist-to-hip ratio [282].

Ginger has been shown to be quite helpful with weight loss. It helps to lower overall bodyweight, it decreases the waist to hip ratio and increases HDL levels [283].

Another way in which ginger helps with fat loss is that it helps to regulate the bacteria that is in the gut. It increases bifidobacteria and other bacteria that make short chain fatty acids (allobaculum & alloprevotella) [284].

The production of fecal short chain fatty acids is a surprisingly important key to preventing and getting rid of belly fat. Short chain fatty acids help to regulate basically everything from gut health to metabolic and immune health. Research has shown that low concentrations of fecal short chain fatty acids is related to higher odds of having central/visceral obesity [285].

NIGELLA SATIVA

Black seed oil or black cumin, also known as nigella sativa, is a plant that has been used medicinally for a lot of different conditions. The oil is more effective than the powder, so black seed oil has become a popular health supplement. However, simply taking the crushed seeds can yield great results especially when working synergistically with aerobic exercise. One study showed that doing this caused its participants to have lower total and LDL cholesterol, lower overall BMI, and lower triglycerides [286]. Doing it this way also helped to increase HDL cholesterol and even assisted with improving their V02 max levels [287]. Black cumin can be taken in different ways, and when taking as a supplement (NOT cooking), the oil has been found to be a potent healer.

Black seed oil helps improve liver enzymes in people who have fatty liver disease. It also helps with insulin resistance and high blood sugar [288].

It's effective at reducing total bodyweight and waist circumference, [289] it reduces toxic visceral fat and reduces overall body fat percentage while making the body have a healthier reaction to food, doing a better job at recognizing when it is satisfied at the end of meals [290].

TURMERIC

Turmeric is a powerful antioxidant root that is often used to make Indian cuisine, weight loss drinks, dye fabric, and simply taken as a supplement. Many people who have heard of turmeric have heard of curcumin as well, but they are not exactly the same. They come from the same plant, but curcumin is the yellow carotenoid that gives turmeric root its yellow hue. Both can be taken as a supplement but turmeric is less processed and less isolated than curcumin.

Both turmeric and curcumin have been shown to reduce body fat percentage as well as waist circumference [291]. They also help to balance different hormones in the body by increasing levels of adiponectin and also by increasing the satiety hormone, leptin [292].

This is another supplement that can be taken to lessen the negative effects of cheat meals. It helps to reduce the amount of visceral fat that accumulates while under a high fat diet [293]. While helpful, there is a drawback, it can also increase oxidative stress.

As for those who have PCOS, curcumin can be quite impactful. It reduced DHT hormone levels, increased estradiol and also reduced the fasting glucose levels without any negative effects [294].

Now that you have information on a lot of supplements that have been proven to help get rid of belly fat, you can use it at your and your doctors discretion. Remember that the most effective way to benefit out of this to include this in your total lifestyle change, though. Taking a supplement can help, but it's not going to be the total answer.

Adding supplements to your routine can help a lot when you're having your cheat meals, it could help to lessen the negative effects, and you may not even experience the added pounds or inches to your waist if you include them on the days/times you have your cheat meals. This can make it so much easier to bounce back. Supplements can be a bonus, but do not rely on them because without an overall healthy lifestyle, supplements will not be enough.

Chapter Twenty-One

Your emotions influence your waist size

S tress and emotions can have an effect on our health, resulting in us developing wider waistlines, so it's important to know how to deal with stress. It's important to improve your stress levels in a meaningful and impactful way, rather than just managing your stress in an unproductive and ineffective way. Doing something about your stress is important because our minds have real effects on our bodies. When you have a stressful situation, it has to be truly dealt with, not ignored.

Stress *is* a normal part of life, but sometimes it gets out of hand. There's good stress and bad stress, and you guessed it, the *bad* kind negatively affects your waistline.According to the American Psychological Association, stress is **"any uncomfortable emotional experience accompanied by predictable biochemical, physiological and behavioral changes"** [295]. The most important solution to stress, is to *add positive emotions* in the mix [296], because if *all* you have is negative emotions, you're on a serious downward spiral. Think of stress as a math problem. When bad stress is high, good feelings need to be added. Stress may, at times, be something that we cannot remove, but your mental health can benefit by adding positive emotions in to your life.

Stress affects the human body in several ways. When you feel stressed, your body creates a hormone called cortisol. This hormone works with your body to control the moods: ***motivation*** **and** ***fear***. Cortisol itself isn't all bad, it can actually be health-promoting (motivational). Cortisol is also used for bodily functions, like the management of carbohydrates, fats, and proteins [297].

Cortisol is also able to keep inflammation levels down, regulate blood pressure, control your sleep/wake cycle, and boost energy levels [298] so that you can handle your responsibilities (eustress).

When your body is ***too*** **stressed** and it's ***over-exposed*** **to cortisol** from fear and negative emotions, the processes in your body become disrupted and **cortisol becomes** ***destructive***. This is why cortisol has been associated with larger waistlines and disease.

According to the American Psychological Association, negative emotions like **anger, fear, and depression** are *reliably* associated with **poorer health** [299]. In fact, simply having depression can actually be the reason why your waistline is not where you want it to be.

Depression, according to Frontiers in Neuroscience, is a highly prevalent mood disorder in modern society and is associated with significant impairments in a person's quality of life [300].

There is also evidence that psychological stress can activate the *inflammatory response,* which as you now know, causes larger waistlines [301][302].

That means that allowing negative emotions to take up your time and energy will not help you to get the waistline you desire.

This may sound super discouraging, but there's a way to turn it around. You have to **look for experiences** and **think of things** that make you feel **positive emotions.** You have to revisit and retranslate your negative experiences and transform your negative perspectives into something less negative and more positive. Find your happiness by mentally flipping the script. When we have positive emotions, they contribute to achieving a healthy mind and as a result, a healthy waistline [303]. A healthy mind is so valuable because **our bodies and our minds are interconnected.**

According to the American Psychological Association, **greater diversity in day-to-day positive emotions** was associated with **lower levels of inflammation** in circulation within the body [304]. That means that the more variety of positive emotions you encourage yourself to have, the better. This could be **excitement, anticipation, gratefulness, kindness, generosity, relaxation and more.**

Don't let your negative emotions get the best of you! If there's an issue that needs resolving, have the courage to do what's hard, and begin your new life experience because your health is at stake. Do what you know is best for your happiness. Introduce truly positive and uplifting experiences in your life that would help cheer you up and at the same time eliminate negative experiences from your life that you know that you have control over.

Release trying to control situations that are not in your control. Find a good book to read, spend time with people who make you laugh and feel good, go on an adventure, make new friends that have similar goals/dreams and learn how to deal with difficult people in a way that preserves your peace of mind.

Sometimes we experience really stressful times, but that same energy that we use to ruminate/obsess over and keep revisiting stressful thoughts can be put towards having positive thoughts and experiences and connecting with others. It really is a matter of our health, and your waistline will repay you, too.

Maybe this sounds like a lot to change, and maybe you don't know where to start. So here are 5 practical steps to lower your stress levels:

When people say things like "manage your stress," it starts to sound like stress is just something that you have to live with, rather than something that you can reduce. But it isn't as hopeless as people make it out to be. Stress *can* be reduced, it just takes some thinking and some action. So consider these 5 steps to help you reduce your stress:

1. **Decide what you want in life**

What kind of life do you want to live? Let your imagination create a visual depiction of what that life looks like. When you know what you want in life, it makes it clearer how much work needs to be done to get there. While this may seem discouraging, it is necessary to find out what you want in order to get started on the path towards actually living that life. Make this dream your goal.

2. **Consider the reality of the situation**

Reflect on the current state of your life and decide whether there are habits in your life that *help you* **towards** your goal *or discourage you* **from** your goal. The more honest you can be with yourself about your current situation, the better. Get to the root of what is stressing you out and assess how much control you have over the situation.

3. Figure it out - Make a plan, take action

So at this point you should know what you can control and what is out of your control. Focus on what you can control. Be willing to make major changes to your life in order to get closer to the life that you want. Think outside of the box to solutions that you may have not considered before. Remember that **you** are the one who has to make it happen, so take responsibility and get started. Realize that if you do a little bit each day, you're creating **a state of hope** for yourself.

4. Accept the outcome

You may have to make some sacrifices. For example: a break up, paying a lot of money, or giving up your favorite foods for awhile. Sometimes we have to make sacrifices to live the life we want and to experience a higher level of happiness. In this case there is mental work to do: to **accept the negative processes because the positive outcomes are worth** more.

Get yourself in a mental state to do what's necessary in order to reduce your stress. Make friends and develop closer relationships with people who want to live similarly or are already living a life like the one you'd like to live. Find a balance between setting boundaries with those who are not helpful and being the one who shares the life you choose to live by inviting others to do it with you. Mindset is everything, so for the things that you cannot control, remember to explore more positive, yet realistic mental perspectives around those situations. Being positive doesn't mean that you have to lie to yourself or be unrealistic. If you don't enjoy exercising, you don't have to lie to yourself. You can be positive about the benefits that you *do* enjoy that arise from exercising, like feeling good afterwards, feeling proud of yourself, or just the enjoyment of getting fresh air.

5. Make sure to have fun all along the way

If you're so regimented and structured that you leave out fun and relaxation, you're being too hard on yourself. It is admittedly difficult to maintain a strict lifestyle without feeling some degree of stress. And since we are talking about reducing stress here, fun and play are essential to add to your regimen.

You're not a robot, you're a human being who needs a healthy balance. Remember to have fun and take breaks. How can you expect to embrace such a drastic change if you do not take the time to unwind? **Find ways to unwind that align with your new lifestyle, and you'll really see progress.**

I hope these steps are helpful with whatever situation you're in that is a major source of your stress. We have real issues, and while deep breathing, meditation, and venting to friends may be useful, we have to get down to the root of our issues so that we can take action to actually fix them. Then, instead of just managing our stress, we can truly say that we *got rid* of some stress.

If these tips don't work for you, or if you feel you need serious help, don't be afraid to get help. Consulting a therapist could be exactly what you need, so don't stand in your own way, reach out to a therapist.

Chapter Twenty-Two

Mental strength, managing cravings and self control tips

I n society, we're going to run into people, go to events, and we'll even pass by places that tempt us to put our goals lower on our priority list, trading them for things that only make us suffer from poorer health later on.

This chapter will empower you to make decisions that line up with your goals, even when temptation is at its strongest.

Cravings are the worst and most difficult hurdle when switching to a healthy diet. And by cravings, I mean when you're strongly desiring to eat something that you are not supposed to be eating.

Refusing to eat something you want is difficult *in the beginning*. So for those rough times when you're craving something or when you're being offered something that you know that you shouldn't eat, try this. This technique works when other techniques won't:

Remember how it makes you feel afterwards

Just about everyone has some symptom that gets aggravated when they eat junk food. What is your symptom? Do you get tired? Constipated? Develop acne? Insomnia? Bloating? Remind yourself of this consequence. The reality is, you're not rewarding yourself by eating unhealthy food, you're making your future worse. You're taking a little reward for the moment, only to sacrifice true satisfaction over time. Eating bad may feel good in the moment, but an ever-expanding waist and declining health feels terrible. Remember that all you need to do is stay dedicated for awhile to see the results that you desire. It ends up being a worthwhile trade: trading short-lived experiences for long-term success isn't much of a sacrifice in the end.

Remind yourself that this craving is just a feeling that will go away

All you have to do is hold on. It could take as little as 2 weeks to as much as 3 months depending on what your lifestyle was like before and how you made the switch. For me, my cravings go away completely within a month of strict healthy eating. All you have to do is be strong for a time, then the cravings will go away NATURALLY. I often tell myself that I can revisit the unhealthy food later, and then I end up not revisiting it for longer than I thought that I could.

Remember that if you don't practice a healthy lifestyle, nobody will make you do it.

You could choose to eat hot dogs every day or sneak eating candy in the middle of the night and *no one could really stop you*. Ultimately it comes down to self control. Nobody can force you to be healthy or support you at all times that you feel you need support. When we start making our own food choices, essentially **we become our own parents**. We just have to get into the practice of telling ourselves "no," and *obeying ourselves*. Because ultimately your life is up to you, and you alone.

Focus on finding healthy food that's tasty *to you*.

When cravings come, a lot of the time it's because you are hungry or thirsty. So eat *something healthy* or drink some water or tea. Having healthy snacks on hand in the beginning of your lifestyle transition will be advantageous, and will keep you from giving into temptation. Slowly the strong feeling of temptation will fade into nothing. Cravings won't have as much power over you.

Lastly, remember to **claim your future**.

Cravings are temporary and so is your body. It's time that we learn to treasure our bodies and to stop trading temporary joys for our health.

Don't give your health away for a craving that won't even stay. You made a plan to do this, and you're going to be able to do it. You'll be able to live life the way you want, it just takes commitment to this change.

Find a More Meaningful Way to Bond

There is a common belief that food is a perfect way to bond with friends or family. However, if you're on your way to a fit, healthy body, bonding over food is not the best option. Not very many people in this world are committed to being healthy on a consistent basis. Eating healthy and exercising requires enormous effort and willpower and that's when bonding over food can be tricky.

Trying to get closer to your relatives or friends over lunch or dinner can pull you off the path to better health and a healthy waist size. When food is made to be the main event or the main way to have fun, health often gets thrown out the door. But let's just say you have to be at an event like this and it isn't your time to have a cheat meal. It would be extremely hard for you to watch your close friends or family eating your favorite foods, snacks, desserts, and fried and processed food. The temptation to take a bite or to order the same options for yourself can feel irresistible. This is why you have to **be an active part of the change in our culture**.

Make sure to plan healthy events and get-togethers, invite friends and family to healthy food events, or even plan activities that have nothing to do with food but are centered instead around activities that are active, like **5k races, playing tennis, rock climbing, or getting manicures and pedicures**. Every time you meet with a friend of family member doesn't have to be when it's time to eat.

Invite your friends for **morning yoga** or **jogging**, organize a **bicycle ride**, invite your family to an **exercise class**, do a **pottery class** with your friends and **go to a salad place** afterwards. Be the role model that your friends and family need. Create a safe place for friends and family that want to be healthy, too.

You'd be surprised how many people *want* to be in an environment that allows them to lose weight easily too. Show everyone that being fit and eating healthy can be filled with fun activities, too.

Inspire, recruit and **motivate** other people by being an example to others, and never cease working towards your goal. You are strong enough to make it happen. You know how much influence your family and friends have had on you - for better or for worse - so make a conscious and intentional effort to be a part of the culture that influences society to be healthier, all while having fun.

So now you know that you can **be the influence, rather than be influenced** and that becoming a positive health influence is a necessary part of your transformation - because relationships are real and they do have their effects. It's like in sports where there's a defense and an offense. If you don't have a good offense, then all you have is defense, but if you have both, then it can make you extremely powerful and unstoppable.

You may be wondering, "Is this going to be a struggle?" or "Can I find happiness in this new lifestyle?"

Everything you've tried and failed at and tried again has been something that was **very important to you**. If it weren't important, you wouldn't have gotten back up to try again.

Goals.

Goals are everything to us. They're what drives us to keep going, what drives us to take action, what floods our minds with worry and obsession.

Goals are in essence, **our ideal life**. We want ultimate happiness, and we have desires for our future.

Even when we're accomplishing the little daily goals, we feel significantly better. And research has confirmed this to be true: pursuing life-improving goals really does result in more happiness [305]. It's like when you don't want to go to the gym, but then after you forced yourself to go, you feel GOOD. Life just flows after that, things feel easier, better.

That's because we stuck to the plan, and that is *extremely rewarding*.

You begin to believe in yourself and you begin to be able to *trust yourself* to do the thing that you said you were going to do.

You grow more confident in your capabilities and you even begin liking yourself more than before. There's no question as to whether this lifestyle is one in which you can find happiness.

You've already decided your goals, because **where every misery lies, are goals that we never got to achieve**. When we give up on our goals we begin to die, because happiness is life, and sadness is death. Achieved goals are like small deposits of happiness and emotional stability in your mind.

So keep up the good work, or get started back on it again! It's time to really live life. The sooner you get started, the better.

Past Decisions Don't Define Your Future

Reaching goals can sometimes be a path that isn't that clear cut.

We have bumps along the way and sometimes we have to do things differently. Sometimes the only thing in the way is the way that we are thinking:

Our perspective.

It's super important to be able to come up with a way of thinking that will help you to maintain this lifestyle because when you're done with this book, **it'll be up to you** to stay consistent.

How to Grow in Consistency - Don't be Hard on Yourself:

Have you ever eaten so much junky food that you decided that you may as well start eating healthy on Monday or next week/month? As though the failure was so bad that you began to define yourself as a failure who *isn't ready* for change? That maybe you need a few more days before you can start all over again?

That's the discouragement trap. When you're thinking that you need this and that you need that in order to accomplish your goals. <u>Ultimately it makes you play the waiting game</u>. Wait until **next week, next month, next year**. So at first you *thought* you were failing, but now you're **actually failing**. And it only causes you to think that you are less and less capable.

But you *are* capable, and maybe you shouldn't view it as failure.

Sometimes we eat unhealthy food.

Sometimes we make certain purposeful decisions or sometimes we make mistakes. Maybe you're on vacation, maybe you just feel like it.

Every new moment is a new opportunity to do something different. You don't have to be stuck in a state where you can't improve/progress.

Ultimately it is a decision. And taking ownership of that fact that you decided to break the rules, is actually empowering because you can make a different decision *whenever you want*. You can choose to make decisions that are in opposition to your goals or you can choose to make decisions that fulfill your goals.

There's a certain lifestyle that comes with a healthy waist size, and knowing that, is what you'll want to keep in mind whenever you make a decision for better or worse. Next step is to make a choice to always be winning. It's simple math. Always be making progress. This is about feeling good and always knowing in the back of your mind, that you're still reaching your goals.

Know what type of person you want to be, what type of life you want to live, and **make that lifestyle take up the larger percentage of what you do.** Either way you will be accomplishing a goal rather than working against the goal. It's all about mindset and it's in your control.

So this works well for choosing the right type of food to eat, but when it comes to exercise, sometimes it feels like you can't help but have difficulty staying consistent with exercise. It can feel like it isn't in your control to fail when it comes to exercising:

The Importance of a Sustainable Plan

Pushing yourself is an important and necessary thing to do but sometimes it can go too far and backfire. Have you ever been exercising and you kept trying to convince yourself that **what you were doing was not enough**, that you needed to go faster, harder, do more? Well that's what I'm referring to, there needs to be a **healthy balance** when it comes to *how far* and *how often* you push yourself.

This all goes back to the story of the tortoise and the hare. The tortoise was slow and steady, while the hare raced as fast as it could. But, of course, slow and steady wins the race.

The point is that it's the same with exercise. It's more about being **consistent**, than it is about going hard and exercising intensely. Our bodies need to be able to manage weekly and monthly amounts of exercise, and if we are pushing too hard, it will be nearly impossible to stay consistent because *our bodies will **make** us rest at some point.*

Signs you are probably pushing too hard:

1. You can't exercise or eat healthy consistently

2. You go through phases of binging on food to make up for all the energy you used up during that really intense workout last week

3. You lie around being lazy, also known as recuperating

4. You're mentally hard on yourself

5. You feel unprepared to start again mentally or physically

If any of these apply to you, you may be pushing yourself too hard. In order to break the cycle, you have to lighten up on yourself.

You are not someone that can be controlled, you have to find out what makes you tick, what works for you, to be reasonable with yourself.

Find something that you can do consistently and daily, something that you enjoy. Here are some things that can help you to get back on track:

Focus on consistency: It's easier to do 2 miles a day for 3 days, than to do 6 miles every 3 days. 6 miles is a lot to do in one day and that can be exhausting. It's easier to walk 30 minutes every day than to jog 30 minutes every day. Do something that you know your body will be able to handle without causing issues for you. And trust that your body will prepare itself to handle more exercise, in its own time.

Figure out a workout/diet plan that you know you can do on a daily basis, one that is easy, yet also challenging enough. For example, Janey walks about 2.5 miles daily 5 days a week with a walking group that she started. She also does bodyweight exercises once or twice a week depending on how she recuperates and refuels throughout the week. That way, she is able to be more consistent and more motivated to exercise consistently from week to week.

Find something fun: Do something that accomplishes a fitness goal, like joining a local sports league or dance class. Remember that when you mix your goals with something fun, it makes it easy to stay committed and will help it to feel less like work. When exercise is fun, it is easier to stay consistent. If you constantly dread exercising, then you will consistently avoid it, so make sure it is something that makes you excited and happy. An example of this is that when Robby gets off work each day, instead of taking the train home he uses his rollerblades.

Redefine yourself

Why does it always seem like when challenges end, we go back to our old ways of doing things? Because we viewed it as a challenge, and not **who we are**.

Your whole way of thinking has to change in order to make a change final.

It isn't possible to change your lifestyle without experiencing **inner change**. If there are things about a healthy lifestyle that you can't see yourself doing for the next 10 years, *realize that behavior change isn't the key, mental change is.*

Learning to embrace what's healthy and to view it in a positive light are major keys to making a lifestyle change that you can maintain for the long term.

Think of why you bought this book. What were the difficulties that you were dealing with? Do you still want the negative things associated with your old life? If not, then you have to maintain this change, for you. Sure, you may want to indulge every now and then, who doesn't? But now you know better, and you know that a lot of it is in your control.

You know how to gain weight and you know how to lose it, you know how to improve your lifestyle and you know how to destroy it.

Just remember your worth.

Ask yourself: **what would my future self be happy with?**

What can I do today that my future self would thank me for?

Now you are well-equipped to lose your belly fat, and it all boils down to health.

It isn't all about outer body goals, but about **inner body goals**.

We can't have the outer appearance right without the inner body being right.

Lastly, keep close the people you've met (and continue to meet) who have the same desire to be healthy. Always be the person who suggests something active and healthy. Change is the hardest part, but once you've changed, it just feels *normal, natural, and right.* So embrace the benefits of this lifestyle and let go of the drawbacks of your old lifestyle.

Now you're equipped with the information that you need to reach your body goals. It's up to you what you do with it.

I hope that you're feeling much more prepared and excited for your health journey ahead, and I wish you great success in reaching your health and fitness body goals, and remember I'm here for you and your success.

1. Ford ES, Maynard LM, Li C. Trends in Mean Waist Circumference and Abdominal Obesity Among US Adults, 1999-2012. JAMA. 2014;312(11):1151–1153. doi:10.1001/jama.2014. 8362

2. Fauziana, R., Jeyagurunathan, A., Abdin, E., Vaingankar, J. A., Sagayadevan, V., Shafie, S., Sambasivam, R., Chong, S. A., & Subramaniam, M. (2016). Body mass index, waist-hip ratio and risk of chronic medical condition in the elderly population: results from the Well-being of the Singapore Elderly (WiSE) Study. BMC Geriatrics, 16(1). https://doi.or g/10.1186/s12877-016-0297-z

3. Srikanthan, P., Seeman, T. E., & Karlamangla, A. S. (2009). Waist-Hip-Ratio as a predictor of All-Cause mortality in High-Functioning Older Adults. *Annals of Epidemiology, 19*(10), 724–731. https://doi .org/10.1016/j.annepidem.2009.05.003

4. Flegal, K. Waist circumference of healthy men and women in the United States. Int J Obes 31, 1134–1139 (2007). https://doi.org/10.1038/sj.ijo. 0803566

5. Ford, E.S., Mokdad, A.H. and Giles, W.H. (2003), Trends in Waist Circumference among U.S. Adults. Obesity Research, 11: 1223-1231. https://doi.org/10.1038/oby.2003.168 https://onlinelibrary .wiley.com/doi/epdf/10.1038/oby.2003.168

6. Ford ES, Maynard LM, Li C. Trends in Mean Waist Circumference and Abdominal Obesity Among US Adults, 1999-2012. JAMA. 2014;312(11):1151–1153. doi:10.1001/jama.2014.8362 https://jamane twork.com/journals/jama/fullarticle/1904816

7. Sun JY, Huang WJ, Hua Y, Qu Q, Cheng C, Liu HL, Kong XQ, Ma YX, Sun W. Trends in general and abdominal obesity in US adults: Evidence from the National Health and Nutrition Examination Survey (2001-2018). Front Public Health. 2022 Oct 6;10:925293. doi: 10.338 9/fpubh.2022.925293. PMID: 36276394; PMCID: PMC9582849. Retrieved from https://www.ncbi.nlm.nih.gov/pmc/articles/PMC958284 9/

8. Koster, et al 2008, Koster, A., Leitzmann, M. F., Schatzkin, A., Mouw, T., Adams, K. F., Van Eijk, J. T., . . . Harris, T. B. (2008). Waist Circumference and Mortality. American Journal of Epidemiology, 167(12), 1465-1475. Retrieved from https://academic.oup.com/aje/article/167/12/1465/89 017

9. Jacobs, E. J., Newton, C. C., Wang, Y., Patel, A. V., McCullough, M. L., Campbell, P. T., Thun, M. J., & Gapstur, S. M. (2010). Waist circumference and All-Cause mortality in a large US cohort. Archives of Internal Medicine, 170(15), 1293. https://doi.org/10.1001/archinternmed.2010 .201

10. Arsenault, B. J., Lemieux, I., Després, J., Wareham, N. J., Kastelein, J. J., Khaw, K., & Boekholdt, S. M. (2010). The hypertriglyceridemic-waist phenotype and the risk of coronary artery disease: results from the EPIC-Norfolk Prospective Population Study. Canadian Medical Association Journal, 182(13), 1427–1432. https://doi.org/10.1503/cmaj.091276

11. Arsenault, B. J., Lemieux, I., Després, J., Wareham, N. J., Kastelein, J. J., Khaw, K., & Boekholdt, S. M. (2010). The hypertriglyceridemic-waist phenotype and the risk of coronary artery disease: results from the EPIC-Norfolk Prospective Population Study. Canadian Medical Association Journal, 182(13), 1427–1432. https://doi.org/10.1503/cmaj.091276

12. Hermsdorff, H.H.M., Zulet, M.Á., Puchau, B. et al. Central Adiposity Rather Than Total Adiposity Measurements Are Specifically Involved in the Inflammatory Status from Healthy Young Adults. Inflammation 34, 161–170 (2011). https://doi.org/10.1007/s10753-010-9219 -y

13. David G Carey, Arthur B Jenkins, Lesley V Campbell, Judith Freund, Donald J Chisholm; Abdominal Fat and Insulin Resistance in Normal and Overweight Women: Direct Measurements Reveal a Strong Relationship in Subjects at Both Low and High Risk of NIDDM. Diabetes 1 May 1996; 45 (5): 633–638. https://doi.org/10.2337/diab.45.5.633

14. Manolopoulos KN, Karpe F, Frayn KN. Gluteofemoral body fat as a determinant of metabolic health. Int J Obes (Lond). 2010 Jun;34(6):949-59. doi: 10.1038/ijo.2009.286. Epub 2010 Jan 12. PMID: 20065965. https://www.ncbi.nlm.nih.gov/pubmed/20065965

15. Hermsdorff, H. H. M., Zulet, M. Á., Puchau, B., & Martínéz, J. A. (2010). Central Adiposity Rather Than Total Adiposity Measurements Are Specifically Involved in the Inflammatory Status from Healthy Young Adults. Inflammation, 34(3), 161–170. https://doi.org/10.1007/s10753 -010-9219-y

16. Manolopoulos KN, Karpe F, Frayn KN. Gluteofemoral body fat as a determinant of metabolic health. Int J Obes (Lond). 2010 Jun;34(6):949-59. doi: 10.1038/ijo.2009.286. Epub 2010 Jan 12. PMID: 20065965. https: //www.ncbi.nlm.nih.gov/pubmed/20065965

17. Snijder, M. B., Dekker, J., Visser, M., Yudkin, J., Stehouwer, C. D., Bouter, L. M., Heine, R. J., Nijpels, G., & Seidell, J. C. (2003). Larger Thigh and Hip Circumferences Are Associated with Better Glucose Tolerance: The Hoorn Study. Obesity Research, 11(1), 104–111. https://doi.org/10.10 38/oby.2003.18

18. David G Carey, Arthur B Jenkins, Lesley V Campbell, Judith Freund, Donald J Chisholm; Abdominal Fat and Insulin Resistance in Normal and Overweight Women: Direct Measurements Reveal a Strong Relationship in Subjects at Both Low and High Risk of NIDDM. Diabetes 1 May 1996; 45 (5): 633–638. https://doi.org/10.2337/diab.45.5.633

19. Emanuela Lapice, Simona Maione, Lidia Patti, Paola Cipriano, Angela A. Rivellese, Gabriele Riccardi, Olga Vaccaro; Abdominal Adiposity Is Associated With Elevated C-Reactive Protein Independent of BMI in Healthy Nonobese People. Diabetes Care 1 September 2009; 32 (9): 1734–1736. https://doi.org/10.2337/dc09-0176

20. Ackermann, D., Jones, J., Barona, J., Calle, M. C., Kim, J. E., Lapia, B., ... Fernandez, M. L. (2011). Waist circumference is positively correlated with markers of inflammation and negatively with adiponectin in women with metabolic syndrome. Nutrition Research, 31(3), 197–204. doi: 10.1016 /j.nutres.2011.02.004

21. Panagiotakos, D., Pitsavos, C., Yannakoulia, M., Chrysohoou, C., & Stefanadis, C. (2005). The implication of obesity and central fat on markers of chronic inflammation: The ATTICA study. Atherosclerosis, 183(2), 308–315. doi: 10.1016/j.atherosclerosis.2005.03.010

22. Huang, L., Xue, J., He, Y., Wang, J., Sun, C., Feng, R., Teng, J., He, Y., & Li, Y. (2011). Dietary Calcium but Not Elemental Calcium from Supplements Is Associated with Body Composition and Obesity in Chinese Women. PLOS ONE, 6(12), e27703. https://doi.org/10.1371/journal.p one.0027703

23. Thomas-Valdés, S., Tostes, M. D. G. V., Anunciação, P. C., Da Silva, B. P., & Santana, H. (2017). Association between vitamin deficiency and metabolic disorders related to obesity. Critical Reviews in Food Science and Nutrition, 57(15), 3332–3343. https://doi.org/10.1080/10408398 .2015.1117413

24. Hosseini, B., Saedisomeolia, A., & Allman-Farinelli, M. (2016). Association Between Antioxidant Intake/Status and Obesity: a Systematic Review of Observational Studies. Biological Trace Element Research, 175(2), 287–297. https://doi.org/10.1007/s12011-016-0785-1

25. Goncalves A, Amiot MJ. Fat-soluble micronutrients and metabolic syndrome. Curr Opin Clin Nutr Metab Care. 2017 Nov;20(6):492-497. doi: 10.1097/MCO.0000000000000412. PMID: 28858890; PMCID: PMC5639995. https://www.ncbi.nlm.nih.gov/pmc/articles/PMC5639 995/

26. Silveira, É. A., Ferreira, C., Pagotto, V., De Carvalho Santos, A. S. E. A., & Velásquez-Meléndez, G. (2017b). Total and central obesity in elderly associated with a marker of undernutrition in early life – sitting height-to-stature ratio: A nutritional paradox. American Journal of Human Biology, 29(3). https://doi.org/10.1002/ajhb.22977

27. Pereira, M., De Farias Costa, P. R., Assis, A. M. O., Santos, C. a. S., & Santos, D. B. D. (2015). Obesity and vitamin D deficiency: a systematic review and meta-analysis. Obesity Reviews, 16(4), 341–349. https://doi .org/10.1111/obr.12239

28. Kerns, J. C., Arundel, C., & Chawla, L. S. (2015). Thiamin Deficiency in People with Obesity. Advances in Nutrition, 6(2), 147–153. https://doi .org/10.3945/an.114.007526

29. Suzuki, K., Inoue, T., Hioki, R., Ochiai, J., Kusuhara, Y., Ichino, N., Osakabe, K., Hamajima, N., & Ito, Y. (2006). Association of abdominal obesity with decreased serum levels of carotenoids in a healthy Japanese population. Clinical Nutrition, 25(5), 780–789. https://doi.org/10.101 6/j.clnu.2006.01.025

30. Waniek, S., Di Giuseppe, R., Plachta-Danielzik, S., Ratjen, I., Jacobs, G., Koch, M., Borggrefe, J., Both, M., Müller, H., Kassubek, J., Nöthlings, U., Esatbeyoglu, T., Schlesinger, S., Rimbach, G., & Lieb, W. (2017). Association of Vitamin E Levels with Metabolic Syndrome, and MRI-Derived Body Fat Volumes and Liver Fat Content. Nutrients, 9(10), 1143. https://doi.org/10.3390/nu9101143

31. Samanta Thomas-Valdés, Maria das Graças V. Tostes, Pamella C. Anunciação, Bárbara P. da Silva & Helena M. Pinheiro Sant'Ana (2017) Association between vitamin deficiency and metabolic disorders related to obesity, Critical Reviews in Food Science and Nutrition, 57:15, 3332-3343, DOI: 10.1080/10408398.2015.1117413. https://www.tandfonline.com/doi/abs/10.1080/10408398.2015.1117413

32. Hosseini, B., Saedisomeolia, A. & Allman-Farinelli, M. Association Between Antioxidant Intake/Status and Obesity: a Systematic Review of Observational Studies. Biol Trace Elem Res 175, 287–297 (2017). http s://doi.org/10.1007/s12011-016-0785-1 https://link.springer.com/artic le/10.1007/s12011-016-0785-1

33. Goncalves A, Amiot MJ. Fat-soluble micronutrients and metabolic syndrome. Curr Opin Clin Nutr Metab Care. 2017 Nov;20(6):492-497. doi: 10.1097/MCO.0000000000000412. PMID: 28858890; PMCID: PMC5639995. https://www.ncbi.nlm.nih.gov/pmc/articles/PMC5639 995/

34. Silveira, É. A., Ferreira, C., Pagotto, V., De Carvalho Santos, A. S. E. A., & Velásquez-Meléndez, G. (2017). Total and central obesity in elderly associated with a marker of undernutrition in early life – sitting height-to-stature ratio: A nutritional paradox. American Journal of Human Biology, 29(3). https://doi.org/10.1002/ajhb.22977

35. Kerns JC, Arundel C, Chawla LS. Thiamin deficiency in people with obesity. Adv Nutr. 2015 Mar 13;6(2):147-53. doi: 10.3945/an.114.007526. PMID: 25770253; PMCID: PMC4352173. https://www.ncbi.nlm.nih.gov/pmc/articles/PMC4352173/

36. Suzuki K, Inoue T, Hioki R, Ochiai J, Kusuhara Y, Ichino N, Osakabe K, Hamajima N, Ito Y. Association of abdominal obesity with decreased serum levels of carotenoids in a healthy Japanese population. Clin Nutr. 2006 Oct;25(5):780-9. doi: 10.1016/j.clnu.2006.01.025. Epub 2006 May 15. PMID: 16698146. https://www.ncbi.nlm.nih.gov/pubmed/166981 46

37. Suzuki K, Inoue T, Hioki R, Ochiai J, Kusuhara Y, Ichino N, Osakabe K, Hamajima N, Ito Y. Association of abdominal obesity with decreased serum levels of carotenoids in a healthy Japanese population. Clin Nutr. 2006 Oct;25(5):780-9. doi: 10.1016/j.clnu.2006.01.025. Epub 2006 May 15. PMID: 16698146. https://www.ncbi.nlm.nih.gov/pubmed/166981 46

38. Pereira-Santos M, Costa PR, Assis AM, Santos CA, Santos DB. Obesity and vitamin D deficiency: a systematic review and meta-analysis. Obes Rev. 2015 Apr;16(4):341-9. doi: 10.1111/obr.12239. Epub 2015 Feb 17. PMID: 25688659. https://www.ncbi.nlm.nih.gov/pubmed/25688659

39. Zhang, C., Rexrode, K. M., Van Dam, R. M., Li, T. Y., & Hu, F. B. (2008). Abdominal obesity and the risk of All-Cause, cardiovascular, and cancer mortality. Circulation, 117(13), 1658–1667. https://doi.org/10.1161/ci rculationaha.107.739714

40. Dhawan D, Sharma S. Abdominal Obesity, Adipokines and Non-communicable Diseases. J Steroid Biochem Mol Biol. 2020 Oct;203:105737. doi: 10.1016/j.jsbmb.2020.105737. Epub 2020 Aug 18. PMID: 32818561; PMCID: PMC7431389. Retrieved from https://www.ncbi.nlm.nih.gov/pmc/articles/PMC7431389/.

41. Ylli, D. (2022, September 6). Endocrine changes in obesity. Endotext - NCBI Bookshelf. https://www.ncbi.nlm.nih.gov/books/NBK279053/

42. Wang, X., Ouyang, Y., Liu, J., Zhu, M., Zhao, G., Bao, W., & Hu, F. B. (2014). Fruit and vegetable consumption and mortality from all causes, cardiovascular disease, and cancer: systematic review and dose-response meta-analysis of prospective cohort studies. The BMJ, 349(jul29 3), g4490. https://doi.org/10.1136/bmj.g4490

43. Lydia A. Bazzano, Tricia Y. Li, Kamudi J. Joshipura, Frank B. Hu; Intake of Fruit, Vegetables, and Fruit Juices and Risk of Diabetes in Women. Diabetes Care 1 July 2008; 31 (7): 1311–1317. https://doi.org/10.2337/dc08-0080

44. Fruit and vegetable consumption and mortality from all causes, cardiovascular disease, and cancer: systematic review and dose-response meta-analysis of prospective cohort studies. (2014). The BMJ, 349(sep03 18), g5472. https://doi.org/10.1136/bmj.g5472

45. Fruit and vegetable consumption and mortality from all causes, cardiovascular disease, and cancer: systematic review and dose-response meta-analysis of prospective cohort studies. (2014b). The BMJ, 349(sep03 18), g5472. https://doi.org/10.1136/bmj.g5472

46. Fruit and vegetable consumption and mortality from all causes, cardiovascular disease, and cancer: systematic review and dose-response meta-analysis of prospective cohort studies. (2014). The BMJ, 349(sep03 18), g5472. https://doi.org/10.1136/bmj.g5472

47. Heidemann, C., Schulze, M. B., Franco, O. H., Van Dam, R. M., Mantzoros, C. S., & Hu, F. B. (2008). Dietary patterns and risk of mortality from cardiovascular disease, cancer, and all causes in a prospective cohort of women. Circulation, 118(3), 230–237. https://doi.org/10.1161/circulationaha.108.771881

48. Dawson-Hughes B, Harris SS, Ceglia L. Alkaline diets favor lean tissue mass in older adults. Am J Clin Nutr. 2008 Mar;87(3):662-5. doi: 10.1093/ajcn/87.3.662. PMID: 18326605; PMCID: PMC2597402. https://www.ncbi.nlm.nih.gov/pubmed/18326605

49. Dawson-Hughes B, Harris SS, Ceglia L. Alkaline diets favor lean tissue mass in older adults. Am J Clin Nutr. 2008 Mar;87(3):662-5. doi: 10.1093/ajcn/87.3.662. PMID: 18326605; PMCID: PMC2597402. https://www.ncbi.nlm.nih.gov/pmc/articles/PMC2597402/

50. Orgeron R III, Pope J, Erickson D, Green V. Phytonutrients: A Potential Role in Obesity (P08-047-19). Curr Dev Nutr. 2019 Oct 24;3(Suppl 1):nzz044.P08-047-19. doi: 10.1093/cdn/nzz044.P08-047-19. PMCID: PMC6818905. https://www.ncbi.nlm.nih.gov/pmc/articles/PMC6818905/

51. Cooper, A., Forouhi, N., Ye, Z. et al. Fruit and vegetable intake and type 2 diabetes: EPIC-InterAct prospective study and meta-analysis. Eur J Clin Nutr 66, 1082–1092 (2012). https://doi.org/10.1038/ejcn.2012.85https://www.nature.com/articles/ejcn201285

52. Yan, S., Chen, S., Liu, Y. et al. Associations of serum carotenoids with visceral adiposity index and lipid accumulation product: a cross-sectional study based on NHANES 2001–2006. Lipids Health Dis 22, 209 (2023). https://doi.org/10.1186/s12944-023-01945-6 https://lipidworld.biomedcentral.com/articles/10.1186/s12944-023-01945-6

53. Yao, N., Yan, S., Guo, Y., Wang, H., Li, X., Wang, L., Hu, W., Li, B., & Cui, W. (2021). The association between carotenoids and subjects with overweight or obesity: a systematic review and meta-analysis. Food & Function, 12(11), 4768–4782. https://doi.org/10.1039/d1fo00004g

54. Combet, E., Ma, Z., Cousins, F., Thompson, B., & Lean, M. (2014, July 09). Low-level seaweed supplementation improves iodine status in iodine-insufficient women: British Journal of Nutrition. Retrieved June 05, 2020, from https://www.cambridge.org/core/journals/british-journal-of-nutrition/article/lowlevel-seaweed-supplementation-improves-iodine-status-in-iodineinsufficient-women/E602BCE8ADED587DFA69E7FD86622649

55. Hitoe, S., & Shimoda, H. (2017). Seaweed Fucoxanthin Supplementation Improves Obesity Parameters in Mild Obese Japanese Subjects. Retrieved June 05, 2020, from https://ffhdj.com/index.php/ffhd/article/view/333

56. Kumar, S. A., Magnusson, M., Ward, L. C., Paul, N. A., & Brown, L. (2015, February 02). Seaweed Supplements Normalise Metabolic, Cardiovascular and Liver Responses in High-Carbohydrate, High-Fat Fed Rats. Retrieved June 05, 2020, from https://www.mdpi.com/1660-3397/13/2/788/htm

57. Keast, D. R., O'Neil, C. E., & Jones, J. M. (2011). Dried fruit consumption is associated with improved diet quality and reduced obesity in US adults: National Health and Nutrition Examination Survey, 1999-2004. Nutrition Research, 31(6), 460–467. https://doi.org/10.1016/j.nutres. 2011.05.009

58. Keast, D. R., O'Neil, C. E., & Jones, J. M. (2011). Dried fruit consumption is associated with improved diet quality and reduced obesity in US adults: National Health and Nutrition Examination Survey, 1999-2004. Nutrition Research, 31(6), 460–467. https://doi.org/10.1016/j.nutres. 2011.05.009

59. Pfister R, Sharp SJ, Luben R, Wareham NJ, Khaw KT. Plasma vitamin C predicts incident heart failure in men and women in European Prospective Investigation into Cancer and Nutrition-Norfolk prospective study. Am Heart J. 2011 Aug;162(2):246-53. doi: 10.1016/j.ahj.2011.05.007. Epub 2011 Jul 7. PMID: 21835284. https://www.ncbi.nlm.nih.gov/pubmed/ 21835284

60. McCall DO, McGartland CP, McKinley MC, Patterson CC, Sharpe P, McCance DR, Young IS, Woodside JV. Dietary intake of fruits and vegetables improves microvascular function in hypertensive subjects in a dose-dependent manner. Circulation. 2009 Apr 28;119(16):2153-60. doi: 10.1161/CIRCULATIONAHA.108.831297. Epub 2009 Apr 13. PMID: 19364976. https://www.ncbi.nlm.nih.gov/pubmed/19364976

61. García, O.P., Ronquillo, D., Caamaño, M.d.C. et al. Zinc, vitamin A, and vitamin C status are associated with leptin concentrations and obesity in Mexican women: results from across-sectional study. Nutr Metab (Lond) 9, 59 (2012). https://doi.org/10.1186/1743-7075-9-5 9 https://nutritionandmetabolism.biomedcentral.com/articles/10.1186 /1743-7075-9-59

62. Pfister R, Sharp SJ, Luben R, Wareham NJ, Khaw KT. Plasma vitamin C predicts incident heart failure in men and women in European Prospective Investigation into Cancer and Nutrition-Norfolk prospective study. Am Heart J. 2011 Aug;162(2):246-53. doi: 10.1016/j.ahj.2011.05.007. Epub 2011 Jul 7. PMID: 21835284. https://www.ncbi.nlm.nih.gov/pubmed/ 21835284

63. Anton, S.D., Gallagher, J., Carey, V.J. et al. Diet type and changes in food cravings following weight loss: Findings from the POUNDS LOST Trial. Eat Weight Disord 17, e101–e108 (2012). https://doi.org/10.1007/B F03325333

64. Parker ED, Liu S, Van Horn L, Tinker LF, Shikany JM, Eaton CB, Margolis KL. The association of whole grain consumption with incident type 2 diabetes: the Women's Health Initiative Observational Study. Ann Epidemiol. 2013 Jun;23(6):321-7. doi: 10.1016/j.annepidem.2013.03.010 . Epub 2013 Apr 19. PMID: 23608304; PMCID: PMC3662533. http s://www.ncbi.nlm.nih.gov/pmc/articles/PMC3662533/

65. Jéquier E. Carbohydrates as a source of energy. Am J Clin Nutr. 1994 Mar;59(3 Suppl):682S-685S. doi: 10.1093/ajcn/59.3.682S. PMID: 8116550.

66. Lee Crosby1*, Brenda Davis2, Shivam Joshi3,4, Meghan Jardine1, Jennifer Paul1,5,6, Maggie Neola1 and Neal D. Barnard1,7. Ketogenic Diets and Chronic Disease: Weighing the Benefits Against the Risks. Front. Nutr., 16 July 2021 | https://doi.org/10.3389/fnut.2021.702802

67. McKeown NM, Troy LM, Jacques PF, Hoffmann U, O'Donnell CJ, Fox CS. Whole- and refined-grain intakes are differentially associated with abdominal visceral and subcutaneous adiposity in healthy adults: the Framingham Heart Study. Am J Clin Nutr. 2010 Nov;92(5):1165-71. doi: 10 .3945/ajcn.2009.29106. Epub 2010 Sep 29. PMID: 20881074; PMCID: PMC2954448. https://www.ncbi.nlm.nih.gov/pubmed/20881074

68. Tina Wirström, Agneta Hilding, Harvest F Gu, Claes-Göran Östenson, Anneli Björklund, Consumption of whole grain reduces risk of deteriorating glucose tolerance, including progression to prediabetes, The American Journal of Clinical Nutrition, Volume 97, Issue 1, January 2013, Pages 179–187, https://doi.org/10.3945/ajcn.112.045583

69. Tina Wirström, Agneta Hilding, Harvest F Gu, Claes-Göran Östenson, Anneli Björklund, Consumption of whole grain reduces risk of deteriorating glucose tolerance, including progression to prediabetes, The American Journal of Clinical Nutrition, Volume 97, Issue 1, January 2013, Pages 179–187, https://doi.org/10.3945/ajcn.112.045583

70. https://academic.oup.com/ajcn/article/97/1/179/4577034, Katcher, H., Legro, R. S., Kunselman, A. R., Gillies, P. J., Demers, L. M., Bagshaw, D., & Kris-Etherton, P. M. (2008). The effects of a whole grain–enriched hypocaloric diet on cardiovascular disease risk factors in men and women with metabolic syndrome. The American Journal of Clinical Nutrition, 87(1), 79–90. https://doi.org/10.1093/ajcn/87.1.79

71. Malin, S. K., Kullman, E. L., Scelsi, A. R., Haus, J. M., Filion, J., Pagadala, M., Godin, J., Kochhar, S., Ross, A. B., & Kirwan, J. P. (2018). A whole-grain diet reduces peripheral insulin resistance and improves glucose kinetics in obese adults: A randomized-controlled trial. Metabolism, 82, 111–117. https://doi.org/10.1016/j.metabol.2017.12.011

72. Slavin, J. L. (2010). Whole grains and digestive health. Cereal Chemistry, 87(4), 292–296. https://doi.org/10.1094/cchem-87-4-0292

73. Satya S. Jonnalagadda, Lisa Harnack, Rui Hai Liu, Nicola McKeown, Chris Seal, Simin Liu, George C. Fahey, Putting the Whole Grain Puzzle Together: Health Benefits Associated with Whole Grains—Summary of American Society for Nutrition 2010 Satellite Symposium, The Journal of Nutrition, Volume 141, Issue 5, May 2011, Pages 1011S–1022S, https://doi.org/10.3945/jn.110.132944

74. McKeown NM, Troy LM, Jacques PF, Hoffmann U, O'Donnell CJ, Fox CS. Whole- and refined-grain intakes are differentially associated with abdominal visceral and subcutaneous adiposity in healthy adults: the Framingham Heart Study. Am J Clin Nutr. 2010 Nov;92(5):1165-71. doi: 10.3945/ajcn.2009.29106. Epub 2010 Sep 29. PMID: 20881074; PMCID: PMC2954448

75. Karl, J. P., Meydani, M., Barnett, J. B., Vanegas, S. M., Goldin, B. R., Kane, A., Rasmussen, H., Saltzman, E., Vangay, P., Knights, D., Chen, C. O., Das, S. K., Jonnalagadda, S. S., Meydani, S. N., & Roberts, S. B. (2017). Substituting whole grains for refined grains in a 6-wk randomized trial favorably affects energy-balance metrics in healthy men and postmenopausal women. The American Journal of Clinical Nutrition, 105(3), 589–599. https://doi.org/10.3945/ajcn.116.139683

76. Karl, J. P., Meydani, M., Barnett, J. B., Vanegas, S. M., Goldin, B. R., Kane, A., Rasmussen, H., Saltzman, E., Vangay, P., Knights, D., Chen, C. O., Das, S. K., Jonnalagadda, S. S., Meydani, S. N., & Roberts, S. B. (2017). Substituting whole grains for refined grains in a 6-wk randomized trial favorably affects energy-balance metrics in healthy men and postmenopausal women. The American Journal of Clinical Nutrition, 105(3), 589–599. https://doi.org/10.3945/ajcn.116.139683

77. Satya S. Jonnalagadda, Lisa Harnack, Rui Hai Liu, Nicola McKeown, Chris Seal, Simin Liu, George C. Fahey, Putting the Whole Grain Puzzle Together: Health Benefits Associated with Whole Grains—Summary of American Society for Nutrition 2010 Satellite Symposium, The Journal of Nutrition, Volume 141, Issue 5, May 2011, Pages 1011S–1022S, https://doi.org/10.3945/jn.110.132944

78. Maki KC, Beiseigel JM, Jonnalagadda SS, Gugger CK, Reeves MS, Farmer MV, Kaden VN, Rains TM. Whole-grain ready-to-eat oat cereal, as part of a dietary program for weight loss, reduces low-density lipoprotein cholesterol in adults with overweight and obesity more than a dietary program including low-fiber control foods. J Am Diet Assoc. 2010 Feb;110(2):205-14. doi: 10.1016/j.jada.2009.10.037. PMID: 20102847.

79. Lee, S., Kim, MB., Kim, C. et al. Whole grain cereal attenuates obesity-induced muscle atrophy by activating the PI3K/Akt pathway in obese C57BL/6N mice. Food Sci Biotechnol 27, 159–168 (2018). https://doi.org/10.1007/s10068-017-0277-x

80. StÖPpler, M. C., MD. (2022, July 28). Insulin resistance: Diet, symptoms, treatment, causes, reduce & test. MedicineNet. https://www.medicinenet.com/insulin_resistance/article.htm#what_is_insulin_resistance

81. Malin, S. K., Kullman, E. L., Scelsi, A. R., Haus, J. M., Filion, J., Pagadala, M., Godin, J., Kochhar, S., Ross, A. B., & Kirwan, J. P. (2018b). A whole-grain diet reduces peripheral insulin resistance and improves glucose kinetics in obese adults: A randomized-controlled trial. Metabolism, 82, 111–117. https://doi.org/10.1016/j.metabol.2017.12.011

82. Tina Wirström, Agneta Hilding, Harvest F Gu, Claes-Göran Östenson, Anneli Björklund, Consumption of whole grain reduces risk of deteriorating glucose tolerance, including progression to prediabetes, The American Journal of Clinical Nutrition, Volume 97, Issue 1, January 2013, Pages 179–187, https://doi.org/10.3945/ajcn.112.045583

83. Rueda-Clausen CF, Silva FA, Lindarte MA, et al. Olive, soybean and palm oils intake have a similar acute detrimental effect over the endothelial function in healthy young subjects. Nutr Metab Cardiovasc Dis. 2007;17(1):50-57. doi:10.1016/j.numecd.2005.08.008

84. Li Z, Wong A, Henning SM, et al. Hass avocado modulates postprandial vascular reactivity and postprandial inflammatory responses to a hamburger meal in healthy volunteers. Food Funct. 2013;4(3):384-391. doi :10.1039/c2fo30226h

85. Hamsi, M., Othman, F., Zakaria, Z., Subermaniam, K., Jaarin, K., Das, S., . . . Emran, A. (2015). Effect of consumption of fresh and heated virgin coconut oil on the blood pressure and inflammatory biomarkers: An experimental study in Sprague Dawley rats. Retrieved June 05, 2020, from https://www.ajol.info/index.php/bafm/article/view/118328

86. Cahill LE, Pan A, Chiuve SE, et al. Fried-food consumption and risk of type 2 diabetes and coronary artery disease: a prospective study in 2 cohorts of US women and men. Am J Clin Nutr. 2014;100(2):667-675. doi:10.3945/ajcn.114.084129

87. Sayon-Orea, C., Martinez-Gonzalez, M., Gea, A., Flores-Gomez, E., Basterra-Gortari, F., & Bes-Rastrollo, M. (2013, August 06). Consumption of fried foods and risk of metabolic syndrome: The SUN cohort study. Retrieved June 05, 2020, from https://www.sciencedirect.com/science/article/pii/S0261561413002057

88. Sayon-Orea, C., Martinez-Gonzalez, M., Gea, A., Flores-Gomez, E., Basterra-Gortari, F., & Bes-Rastrollo, M. (2013, August 06). Consumption of fried foods and risk of metabolic syndrome: The SUN cohort study. Retrieved June 05, 2020, from https://www.sciencedirect.com/science/article/pii/S0261561413002057

89. Rueda-Clausen CF, Silva FA, Lindarte MA, et al. Olive, soybean and palm oils intake have a similar acute detrimental effect over the endothelial function in healthy young subjects. Nutr Metab Cardiovasc Dis. 2007;17(1):50-57. doi:10.1016/j.numecd.2005.08.008

90. Villela NR, Aguiar LG, Bahia L, Bottino D, Bouskela E. Does endothelial dysfunction correlate better with waist-to-hip ratio than with body mass index or waist circumference among obese patients?. Clinics (Sao Paulo). 2006;61(1):53-58. doi:10.1590/s1807-59322006000100010

91. Brook RD, Bard RL, Rubenfire M, Ridker PM, Rajagopalan S. Usefulness of visceral obesity (waist/hip ratio) in predicting vascular endothelial function in healthy overweight adults. Am J Cardiol. 2001;88(11):1264-1269. doi:10.1016/s0002-9149(01)02088-4

92. Villela NR, Aguiar LG, Bahia L, Bottino D, Bouskela E. Does endothelial dysfunction correlate better with waist-to-hip ratio than with body mass index or waist circumference among obese patients?. Clinics (Sao Paulo). 2006;61(1):53-58. doi:10.1590/s1807-59322006000100010

93. Brook RD, Bard RL, Rubenfire M, Ridker PM, Rajagopalan S. Usefulness of visceral obesity (waist/hip ratio) in predicting vascular endothelial function in healthy overweight adults. Am J Cardiol. 2001;88(11):1264-1269. doi:10.1016/s0002-9149(01)02088-4

94. Rueda-Clausen CF, Silva FA, Lindarte MA, et al. Olive, soybean and palm oils intake have a similar acute detrimental effect over the endothelial function in healthy young subjects. Nutr Metab Cardiovasc Dis. 2007;17(1):50-57. doi:10.1016/j.numecd.2005.08.008

95. Cortés B, Núñez I, Cofán M, et al. Acute effects of high-fat meals enriched with walnuts or olive oil on postprandial endothelial function. J Am Coll Cardiol. 2006;48(8):1666-1671. doi:10.1016/j.jacc.2006.06.057

96. Sham Nurul-Iman, B., Kamisah, Y., Saad Qodriyah, H., & Jaarin, K. (2013, June 05). Virgin Coconut Oil Prevents Blood Pressure Elevation and Improves Endothelial Functions in Rats Fed with Repeatedly Heated Palm Oil. Retrieved June 05, 2020, from https://www.hindawi.com/journals/ecam/2013/629329/

97. Sayon-Orea, C., Martinez-Gonzalez, M., Gea, A., Flores-Gomez, E., Basterra-Gortari, F., & Bes-Rastrollo, M. (2013, August 06). Consumption of fried foods and risk of metabolic syndrome: The SUN cohort study. Retrieved June 05, 2020, from https://www.sciencedirect.com/science/article/pii/S0261561413002057

98. Li Z, Wong A, Henning SM, et al. Hass avocado modulates postprandial vascular reactivity and postprandial inflammatory responses to a hamburger meal in healthy volunteers. Food Funct. 2013;4(3):384-391. doi :10.1039/c2fo30226h

99. Li Z, Wong A, Henning SM, et al. Hass avocado modulates postprandial vascular reactivity and postprandial inflammatory responses to a hamburger meal in healthy volunteers. Food Funct. 2013;4(3):384-391. doi :10.1039/c2fo30226h

100. Damasceno NR, Sala-Vila A, Cofán M, et al. Mediterranean diet supplemented with nuts reduces waist circumference and shifts lipoprotein subfractions to a less atherogenic pattern in subjects at high cardiovascular risk. Atherosclerosis. 2013;230(2):347-353. doi:10.1016/j.atherosclerosis.2013.08.014

101. Barre, D. E., Mizier-Barre, K. A., Stelmach, E., Hobson, J., Griscti, O., Rudiuk, A., & Muthuthevar, D. (2012, October 04). Flaxseed Lignan Complex Administration in Older Human Type 2 Diabetics Manages Central Obesity and Prothrombosis-An Invitation to Further Investigation into Polypharmacy Reduction. Retrieved June 05, 2020, from https://www.hindawi.com/journals/jnme/2012/585170/

102. Martínez-González MA, Bes-Rastrollo M. Nut consumption, weight gain and obesity: Epidemiological evidence. Nutr Metab Cardiovasc Dis. 2011;21 Suppl 1:S40-S45. doi:10.1016/j.numecd.2010.11.005

103. Damasceno NR, Sala-Vila A, Cofán M, et al. Mediterranean diet supplemented with nuts reduces waist circumference and shifts lipoprotein subfractions to a less atherogenic pattern in subjects at high cardiovascular risk. Atherosclerosis. 2013;230(2):347-353. doi:10.1016/j.atherosclerosis.2013.08.014

104. Barre, D. E., Mizier-Barre, K. A., Stelmach, E., Hobson, J., Griscti, O., Rudiuk, A., & Muthuthevar, D. (2012, October 04). Flaxseed Lignan Complex Administration in Older Human Type 2 Diabetics Manages Central Obesity and Prothrombosis-An Invitation to Further Investigation into Polypharmacy Reduction. Retrieved June 05, 2020, from http s://www.hindawi.com/journals/jnme/2012/585170/

105. Barre, D. E., Mizier-Barre, K. A., Stelmach, E., Hobson, J., Griscti, O., Rudiuk, A., & Muthuthevar, D. (2012, October 04). Flaxseed Lignan Complex Administration in Older Human Type 2 Diabetics Manages Central Obesity and Prothrombosis-An Invitation to Further Investigation into Polypharmacy Reduction. Retrieved June 05, 2020, from http s://www.hindawi.com/journals/jnme/2012/585170/

106. Martínez-González MA, Bes-Rastrollo M. Nut consumption, weight gain and obesity: Epidemiological evidence. Nutr Metab Cardiovasc Dis. 2011;21 Suppl 1:S40-S45. doi:10.1016/j.numecd.2010.11.005

107. Damasceno NR, Sala-Vila A, Cofán M, et al. Mediterranean diet supplemented with nuts reduces waist circumference and shifts lipoprotein subfractions to a less atherogenic pattern in subjects at high cardiovascular risk. Atherosclerosis. 2013;230(2):347-353. doi:10.1016/j.atherosclerosi s.2013.08.014

108. Damasceno NR, Sala-Vila A, Cofán M, et al. Mediterranean diet supplemented with nuts reduces waist circumference and shifts lipoprotein subfractions to a less atherogenic pattern in subjects at high cardiovascular risk. Atherosclerosis. 2013;230(2):347-353. doi:10.1016/j.atherosclerosi s.2013.08.014

109. Martínez-González MA, Bes-Rastrollo M. Nut consumption, weight gain and obesity: Epidemiological evidence. Nutr Metab Cardiovasc Dis. 2011;21 Suppl 1:S40-S45. doi:10.1016/j.numecd.2010.11.005

110. Fulgoni, V.L., Dreher, M. & Davenport, A.J. Avocado consumption is associated with better diet quality and nutrient intake, and lower metabolic syndrome risk in US adults: results from the National Health and Nutrition Examination Survey (NHANES) 2001–2008. Nutr J 12, 1 (2013). https://doi.org/10.1186/1475-2891-12-1

111. O'Neil, C.E., Fulgoni, V.L. & Nicklas, T.A. Tree Nut consumption is associated with better adiposity measures and cardiovascular and metabolic syndrome health risk factors in U.S. Adults: NHANES 2005–2010. Nutr J 14, 64 (2015). https://doi.org/10.1186/s12937-015-0052-x. https://nutritionj.biomedcentral.com/articles/10.1186/s12937-015-0052-x

112. Claire E. Berryman, Sheila G. West, Jennifer A. Fleming, Peter L. Bordi and Penny M. Kris-Etherton. Effects of Daily Almond Consumption on Cardiometabolic Risk and Abdominal Adiposity in Healthy Adults With Elevated LDL-Cholesterol: A Randomized Controlled Trial. Originally published5 Jan 2015https://doi.org/10.1161/JAHA.114.000993Journal of the American Heart Association. 2015;4:e000993

113. Santiago, S., Sayón-Orea, C., Babio, N., Ruiz-Canela, M., Martí, A., Corella, D., . . . Martínez, J. (2015, December 12). Yogurt consumption and abdominal obesity reversion in the PREDIMED study. Retrieved June 05, 2020, from https://www.sciencedirect.com/science/article/pii/S0939475315300867

114. Nilsen, R., Hostmark, A. T., Haug, A., & Skeie, S. (2015, August 19). Effect of a high intake of cheese on cholesterol and metabolic syndrome: Results of a randomized trial. Retrieved June 05, 2020, from https://www.tandfonline.com/doi/abs/10.3402/fnr.v59.27651

115. Nilsen, R., Hostmark, A. T., Haug, A., & Skeie, S. (2015, August 19). Effect of a high intake of cheese on cholesterol and metabolic syndrome: Results of a randomized trial. Retrieved June 05, 2020, from https://www.tandfonline.com/doi/abs/10.3402/fnr.v59.27651

116. Nettleton JA, Steffen LM, Loehr LR, Rosamond WD, Folsom AR. Incident heart failure is associated with lower whole-grain intake and greater high-fat dairy and egg intake in the Atherosclerosis Risk in Communities (ARIC) study. J Am Diet Assoc. 2008;108(11):1881-1887. doi:10.1016/j.jada.2008.08.015

117. Crichton GE, Alkerwi A. Whole-fat dairy food intake is inversely associated with obesity prevalence: findings from the Observation of Cardiovascular Risk Factors in Luxembourg study. Nutr Res. 2014;34(11):936-943. doi:10.1016/j.nutres.2014.07.014

118. Van Meijl, L., & Mensink, R. (2010). Effects of low-fat dairy consumption on markers of low-grade systemic inflammation and endothelial function in overweight and obese subjects: An intervention study. British Journal of Nutrition, 104(10), 1523-1527. doi:10.1017/S0007114510002515

119. Koga K, Osuga Y, Tsutsumi O, et al. Increased concentrations of soluble tumour necrosis factor receptor (sTNFR) I and II in peritoneal fluid from women with endometriosis. Mol Hum Reprod. 2000;6(10):929-933. do i:10.1093/molehr/6.10.929

120. Pauline Koh-Banerjee, Nain-Feng Chu, Donna Spiegelman, Bernard Rosner, Graham Colditz, Walter Willett, Eric Rimm, Prospective study of the association of changes in dietary intake, physical activity, alcohol consumption, and smoking with 9-y gain in waist circumference among 16 587 US men, The American Journal of Clinical Nutrition, Volume 78, Issue 4, October 2003, Pages 719–727, https://doi.org/10.1093/ajcn/78.4.719

121. Przybylski O, Aladedunye FA. Formation of trans fats during food preparation. Can J Diet Pract Res. 2012;73(2):98-101. doi:10.3148/73.2.201 2.98

122. Pauline Koh-Banerjee, Nain-Feng Chu, Donna Spiegelman, Bernard Rosner, Graham Colditz, Walter Willett, Eric Rimm, Prospective study of the association of changes in dietary intake, physical activity, alcohol consumption, and smoking with 9-y gain in waist circumference among 16 587 US men, The American Journal of Clinical Nutrition, Volume 78, Issue 4, October 2003, Pages 719–727, https://doi.org/10.1093/ajcn/78.4.719

123. Laura F DeFina, Lucille G Marcoux, Susan M Devers, Joseph P Cleaver, Benjamin L Willis, Effects of omega-3 supplementation in combination with diet and exercise on weight loss and body composition, The American Journal of Clinical Nutrition, Volume 93, Issue 2, February 2011, Pages 455–462, https://doi.org/10.3945/ajcn.110.002741

124. Zhang, Y.Y., Liu, W., Zhao, T.Y. et al. Efficacy of omega-3 polyunsaturated fatty acids supplementation in managing overweight and obesity: A meta-analysis of randomized clinical trials. J Nutr Health Aging 21, 187–192 (2017). https://doi.org/10.1007/s12603-016-0755-5

125. Howe, P.R.C.; Buckley, J.D.; Murphy, K.J.; Pettman, T.; Milte, C.; Coates, A.M. Relationship between Erythrocyte Omega-3 Content and Obesity Is Gender Dependent. Nutrients 2014, 6, 1850-1860.

126. Micallef, M., Munro, I., Phang, M., & Garg, M. (2009). Plasma n-3 polyunsaturated fatty acids are negatively associated with obesity. British Journal of Nutrition, 102(9), 1370-1374. doi:10.1017/S000711450938 2173

127. Benjamin B. Albert, David Cameron-Smith, Paul L. Hofman, Wayne S. Cutfield, "Oxidation of Marine Omega-3 Supplements and Human Health", BioMed Research International, vol. 2013, Article ID 464921, 8 pages, 2013. https://doi.org/10.1155/2013/464921

128. Stephen NM, Jeya Shakila R, Jeyasekaran G, Sukumar D. Effect of different types of heat processing on chemical changes in tuna. J Food Sci Technol. 2010;47(2):174-181. doi:10.1007/s13197-010-0024-2

129. Martins, D., Custódio, L., Barreira, L., Pereira, H., Ben-Hamadou, R., Varela, J., & Abu-Salah, K. (2013, June 27). Alternative sources of n-3 long-chain polyunsaturated fatty acids in marine microalgae. Retrieved June 05, 2020, from https://www.ncbi.nlm.nih.gov/pmc/articles/PMC 3736422/

130. Micallef, M., Munro, I., Phang, M., & Garg, M. (2009). Plasma n-3 polyunsaturated fatty acids are negatively associated with obesity. British Journal of Nutrition, 102(9), 1370-1374. doi:10.1017/S000711450938 2173

131. Micallef, M., Munro, I., Phang, M., & Garg, M. (2009). Plasma n-3 polyunsaturated fatty acids are negatively associated with obesity. British Journal of Nutrition, 102(9), 1370-1374. doi:10.1017/S0007114509382173https://www.cambridge.org/core/jou rnals/british-journal-of-nutrition/article/plasma-n3-polyunsaturated-fatt y-acids-are-negatively-associated-with-obesity/3781A7A37C5CCAA9A B556CC40055814F

132. Halkjær, J., Olsen, A., Overvad, K. et al. Intake of total, animal and plant protein and subsequent changes in weight or waist circumference in European men and women: the Diogenes project. Int J Obes 35, 1104–1113 (2011). https://doi.org/10.1038/ijo.2010.254

133. Freire, R., Fernandes, L., Silva, R. et al. Wheat gluten intake increases weight gain and adiposity associated with reduced thermogenesis and energy expenditure in an animal model of obesity. Int J Obes 40, 479–486 (2016). https://doi.org/10.1038/ijo.2015.204

134. Stefan M Pasiakos, Harris R Lieberman, Victor L Fulgoni, III, Higher-Protein Diets Are Associated with Higher HDL Cholesterol and Lower BMI and Waist Circumference in US Adults, The Journal of Nutrition, Volume 145, Issue 3, March 2015, Pages 605–614, https://doi.org/10.3945/jn.114.205203

135. Weigle DS, Breen PA, Matthys CC, et al. A high-protein diet induces sustained reductions in appetite, ad libitum caloric intake, and body weight despite compensatory changes in diurnal plasma leptin and ghrelin concentrations. Am J Clin Nutr. 2005;82(1):41-48. doi:10.1093/ajcn.82.1.41

136. Yanni Papanikolaou & Victor L. Fulgoni III (2008) Bean Consumption Is Associated with Greater Nutrient Intake, Reduced Systolic Blood Pressure, Lower Body Weight, and a Smaller Waist Circumference in Adults: Results from the National Health and Nutrition Examination Survey 1999-2002, Journal of the American College of Nutrition, 27:5, 569-576, DOI: 10.1080/07315724.2008.10719740

137. Vergnaud AC, Norat T, Romaguera D, et al. Meat consumption and prospective weight change in participants of the EPIC-PANACEA study. Am J Clin Nutr. 2010;92(2):398-407. doi:10.3945/ajcn.2009.28713

138. Tonstad, S., Butler, T., Yan, R., & Fraser, G. (2009, May). Type of vegetarian diet, body weight, and prevalence of type 2 diabetes. Retrieved June 05, 2020, from https://www.ncbi.nlm.nih.gov/pmc/articles/PMC2671114/

139. Wang, Y., & Beydoun, M. A. (2009). Meat consumption is associated with obesity and central obesity among US adults. International Journal of Obesity, 33(6), 621-628. https://doi.org/10.1038/ijo.2009.45

140. Wang, Y., & Beydoun, M. A. (2009). Meat consumption is associated with obesity and central obesity among US adults. International Journal of Obesity, 33(6), 621-628. https://doi.org/10.1038/ijo.2009.45

146

141. Song M, Fung TT, Hu FB, et al. Association of Animal and Plant Protein Intake With All-Cause and Cause-Specific Mortality. JAMA Intern Med. 2016;176(10):1453–1463. doi:10.1001/jamainternmed.2016.4182

142. Wang, Y., & Beydoun, M. A. (2009). Meat consumption is associated with obesity and central obesity among US adults. International Journal of Obesity, 33(6), 621-628. https://doi.org/10.1038/ijo.2009.45

143. Halkjær, J., Olsen, A., Overvad, K. et al. Intake of total, animal and plant protein and subsequent changes in weight or waist circumference in European men and women: the Diogenes project. Int J Obes 35, 1104–1113 (2011). https://doi.org/10.1038/ijo.2010.254

144. Yang, C., Kong, A.P.S., Cai, Z. et al. Persistent Organic Pollutants as Risk Factors for Obesity and Diabetes. Curr Diab Rep 17, 132 (2017). https://doi.org/10.1007/s11892-017-0966-0

145. WHO. (2014, June 20). Persistent organic pollutants (POPs). Retrieved June 05, 2020, from https://www.who.int/foodsafety/areas_work/chemical-risks/pops/en/

146. Barnard, N., Levin, S., & Trapp, C. (2014, February 21). Meat consumption as a risk factor for type 2 diabetes. Retrieved June 05, 2020, from https://www.ncbi.nlm.nih.gov/pmc/articles/PMC3942738/

147. Levine ME, Suarez JA, Brandhorst S, et al. Low protein intake is associated with a major reduction in IGF-1, cancer, and overall mortality in the 65 and younger but not older population. Cell Metab. 2014;19(3):407-417. doi:10.1016/j.cmet.2014.02.006

148. Ponnampalam EN, Mann NJ, Sinclair AJ. Effect of feeding systems on omega-3 fatty acids, conjugated linoleic acid and trans fatty acids in Australian beef cuts: potential impact on human health. Asia Pac J Clin Nutr. 2006;15(1):21-29.

149. Vasanti S. Malik, Yanping Li, Deirdre K. Tobias, An Pan, Frank B. Hu, Dietary Protein Intake and Risk of Type 2 Diabetes in US Men and Women, American Journal of Epidemiology, Volume 183, Issue 8, 15 April 2016, Pages 715–728, https://doi.org/10.1093/aje/kwv268

150. Bernard J Venn, Tracy Perry, Tim J Green, C. Murray Skeaff, Wendy Aitken, Nicky J Moore, Jim I Mann, Alison J Wallace, John Monro, Alison Bradshaw, Rachel C Brown, Paula M.L Skidmore, Kyle Doel, Kerry O'Brien, Chris Frampton & Sheila Williams (2010) The Effect of Increasing Consumption of Pulses and Wholegrains in Obese People: A Randomized Controlled Trial, Journal of the American College of Nutrition, 29:4, 365-372, DOI: 10.1080/07315724.2010.10719853

151. Zare, R., Heshmati, F., Fallahzadeh, H., & Nadjarzadeh, A. (2014, October 13). Effect of cumin powder on body composition and lipid profile in overweight and obese women. Retrieved June 05, 2020, from https://www.sciencedirect.com/science/article/abs/pii/S1744388114000668

152. Lv Jun, Qi Lu, Yu Canqing, Yang Ling, Guo Yu, Chen Yiping et al. Consumption of spicy foods and total and cause specific mortality: population based cohort study BMJ 2015; 351 :h3942

153. Janssens, P., Hursel, R., & Westerterp-Plantenga, M. (2014, March 12). Capsaicin increases sensation of fullness in energy balance, and decreases desire to eat after dinner in negative energy balance. Retrieved June 05, 2020, from https://www.sciencedirect.com/science/article/pii/S019566 6314001123

154. Chen, J., Li, L., Li, Y. et al. Activation of TRPV1 channel by dietary capsaicin improves visceral fat remodeling through connexin43-mediated Ca2+ Influx. Cardiovasc Diabetol 14, 22 (2015). https://doi.org/10.118 6/s12933-015-0183-6

155. Per Björntorp (1992) Abdominal Fat Distribution and Disease: An Overview of Epidemiological Data, Annals of Medicine, 24:1, 15-18, DOI: 10.3109/07853899209164140. https://www.ta ndfonline.com/doi/abs/10.3109/07853899209164140

156. Lourenço, S., Oliveira, A. & Lopes, C. The effect of current and lifetime alcohol consumption on overall and central obesity. Eur J Clin Nutr 66, 813–818 (2012). https://doi.org/10.1038/ejcn.2012.20

157. Vadstrup, E., Petersen, L., Sørensen, T. et al. Waist circumference in relation to history of amount and type of alcohol: results from the Copenhagen City Heart Study. Int J Obes 27, 238–246 (2003). https://doi.org /10.1038/sj.ijo.802203

158. Vadstrup, E., Petersen, L., Sørensen, T. et al. Waist circumference in relation to history of amount and type of alcohol: results from the Copenhagen City Heart Study. Int J Obes 27, 238–246 (2003). https://doi.org /10.1038/sj.ijo.802203

159. TS Han, FCH Bijnen, MEJ Lean, JC Seidell, Separate associations of waist and hip circumference with lifestyle factors, International Journal of Epidemiology, Volume 27, Issue 3, June 1998, Pages 422–430, https://doi.org/10.1093/ije/27.3.422https://academic.oup.com/ije/article/27/3/422/625372

160. Vadstrup, E., Petersen, L., Sørensen, T. et al. Waist circumference in relation to history of amount and type of alcohol: results from the Copenhagen City Heart Study. Int J Obes 27, 238–246 (2003). https://doi.org /10.1038/sj.ijo.802203

161. TS Han, FCH Bijnen, MEJ Lean, JC Seidell, Separate associations of waist and hip circumference with lifestyle factors, International Journal of Epidemiology, Volume 27, Issue 3, June 1998, Pages 422–430, https://doi.org/10.1093/ije/27.3.422

162. Lourenço, S., Oliveira, A. & Lopes, C. The effect of current and lifetime alcohol consumption on overall and central obesity. Eur J Clin Nutr 66, 813–818 (2012). https://doi.org/10.1038/ejcn.2012.20

163. Lourenço, S., Oliveira, A. & Lopes, C. The effect of current and lifetime alcohol consumption on overall and central obesity. Eur J Clin Nutr 66, 813–818 (2012). https://doi.org/10.1038/ejcn.2012.20

164. TS Han, FCH Bijnen, MEJ Lean, JC Seidell, Separate associations of waist and hip circumference with lifestyle factors, International Journal of Epidemiology, Volume 27, Issue 3, June 1998, Pages 422–430, https://doi.org/10.1093/ije/27.3.422

165. Lukasiewicz, E., Mennen, L., Bertrais, S., Arnault, N., Preziosi, P., Galan, P., & Hercberg, S. (2005). Alcohol intake in relation to body mass index and waist-to-hip ratio: The importance of type of alcoholic beverage. Public Health Nutrition, 8(3), 315-320. doi:10.1079/PHN2004680

166. Christiane Bode, J Christian Bode. Effect of alcohol consumption on the gut. Best Practice & Research Clinical Gastroenterology, Volume 17, Issue 4, 2003, Pages 575-592, ISSN 1521-6918. https://doi.org/10.1016/S152 1-6918(03)00034-9.

167. Lukasiewicz, E., Mennen, L., Bertrais, S., Arnault, N., Preziosi, P., Galan, P., & Hercberg, S. (2005). Alcohol intake in relation to body mass index and waist-to-hip ratio: The importance of type of alcoholic beverage. Public Health Nutrition, 8(3), 315-320. doi:10.1079/PHN2004680

168. German JB, Walzem RL. The health benefits of wine. Annu Rev Nutr. 2000;20:561-593. doi:10.1146/annurev.nutr.20.1.561

169. Rod S. Taylor, Kate E. Ashton, Tiffany Moxham, Lee Hooper, Shah Ebrahim, Reduced Dietary Salt for the Prevention of Cardiovascular Disease: A Meta-Analysis of Randomized Controlled Trials (Cochrane Review), American Journal of Hypertension, Volume 24, Issue 8, August 2011, Pages 843–853, https://doi.org/10.1038/ajh.2011.115

170. Rod S. Taylor, Kate E. Ashton, Tiffany Moxham, Lee Hooper, Shah Ebrahim, Reduced Dietary Salt for the Prevention of Cardiovascular Disease: A Meta-Analysis of Randomized Controlled Trials (Cochrane Review), American Journal of Hypertension, Volume 24, Issue 8, August 2011, Pages 843–853, https://doi.org/10.1038/ajh.2011.115

171. Rod S. Taylor, Kate E. Ashton, Tiffany Moxham, Lee Hooper, Shah Ebrahim, Reduced Dietary Salt for the Prevention of Cardiovascular Disease: A Meta-Analysis of Randomized Controlled Trials (Cochrane Review), American Journal of Hypertension, Volume 24, Issue 8, August 2011, Pages 843–853, https://doi.org/10.1038/ajh.2011.115

172. Zhao, L., Daviglus, M., Dyer, A., Horn, L., Garside, D., Zhu, L., . . . Stamler, J. (2012, September 06). Association of Monosodium Glutamate Intake With Overweight in Chinese Adults: The INTERMAP Study. Retrieved June 05, 2020, from https://onlinelibrary.wiley.com/doi/full/10.1038/oby.2008.274

173. Insawang, T., Selmi, C., Cha'on, U. et al. Monosodium glutamate (MSG) intake is associated with the prevalence of metabolic syndrome in a rural Thai population. Nutr Metab (Lond) 9, 50 (2012). https://doi.org/10.1 186/1743-7075-9-50

174. Maria Maersk, Anita Belza, Hans Stødkilde-Jørgensen, Steffen Ring-gaard, Elizaveta Chabanova, Henrik Thomsen, Steen B Peder-sen, Arne Astrup, Bjørn Richelsen, Sucrose-sweetened beverages increase fat storage in the liver, muscle, and visceral fat de-pot: a 6-mo randomized intervention study, The American Journal of Clinical Nutrition, Volume 95, Issue 2, February 2012, Pages 283–289, https://doi.org/10.3945/ajcn.111.022533

175. Kimber L Stanhope, Valentina Medici, Andrew A Bremer, Vivien Lee, Hazel D Lam, Marinelle V Nunez, Guoxia X Chen, Nancy L Keim, Peter J Havel, A dose-response study of consuming high-fruc-tose corn syrup–sweetened beverages on lipid/lipoprotein risk fac-tors for cardiovascular disease in young adults, The American Jour-nal of Clinical Nutrition, Volume 101, Issue 6, June 2015, Pages 1144–1154, https://doi.org/10.3945/ajcn.114.100461

176. Kimber L Stanhope, Valentina Medici, Andrew A Bremer, Vivien Lee, Hazel D Lam, Marinelle V Nunez, Guoxia X Chen, Nancy L Keim, Peter J Havel, A dose-response study of consuming high-fruc-tose corn syrup–sweetened beverages on lipid/lipoprotein risk fac-tors for cardiovascular disease in young adults, The American Jour-nal of Clinical Nutrition, Volume 101, Issue 6, June 2015, Pages 1144–1154, https://doi.org/10.3945/ajcn.114.100461

177. Nseir W, Nassar F, Assy N. Soft drinks consumption and nonalcoholic fatty liver disease. World J Gastroenterol. 2010 Jun 7;16(21):2579-88. doi: 10.3748/wjg.v16.i21.2579. PMID: 20518077; PMCID: PMC2880768.

178. Mathur K, Agrawal RK, Nagpure S, Deshpande D. Effect of artificial sweeteners on insulin resistance among type-2 diabetes mellitus patients. J Family Med Prim Care. 2020 Jan 28;9(1):69-71. doi: 10.4103/jfmpc.j fmpc_329_19. PMID: 32110567; PMCID: PMC7014832. https://ww w.ncbi.nlm.nih.gov/pmc/articles/PMC7014832/

179. Carwile JL, Michels KB. Urinary bisphenol A and obesity: NHANES 2003-2006. Environ Res. 2011;111(6):825-830. doi:10.1016/j.envres.20 11.05.014

180. Wang T, Li M, Chen B, et al. Urinary bisphenol A (BPA) concentration associates with obesity and insulin resistance. J Clin Endocrinol Metab. 2012;97(2):E223-E227. doi:10.1210/jc.2011-1989

181. Ko A, Hwang MS, Park JH, Kang HS, Lee HS, Hong JH. Association between Urinary Bisphenol A and Waist Circumference in Korean Adults. Toxicol Res. 2014;30(1):39-44. doi:10.5487/TR.2014.30.1.039

182. Stahlhut RW, Welshons WV, Swan SH. Bisphenol A data in NHANES suggest longer than expected half-life, substantial nonfood exposure, or both. Environ Health Perspect. 2009 May;117(5):784-9. doi: 10.1289/ehp.0800376. Epub 2009 Jan 28. PMID: 19479022; PMCID: PMC2685842.

183. Arsenault, B., Rana, J., Lemieux, I. et al. Physical inactivity, abdominal obesity and risk of coronary heart disease in apparently healthy men and women. Int J Obes 34, 340–347 (2010). https://doi.org/10.1038/ijo.2009.229

184. Jacobs EJ, Newton CC, Wang Y, et al. Waist Circumference and All-Cause Mortality in a Large US Cohort. Arch Intern Med. 2010;170(15):1293–1301. doi:10.1001/archinternmed.2010.201

185. Nocon M, Hiemann T, Müller-Riemenschneider F, Thalau F, Roll S, Willich SN. Association of physical activity with all-cause and cardiovascular mortality: a systematic review and meta-analysis. Eur J Cardiovasc Prev Rehabil. 2008;15(3):239-246. doi:10.1097/HJR.0b013e3282f55e09

186. CDC. (2017, May 03). FastStats - Deaths and Mortality. Retrieved June 05, 2020, from https://www.cdc.gov/nchs/fastats/deaths.htm

187. **Source: Mortality in the United States, 2021. Data Table for Figure 4. Retrieved from** https://www.cdc.gov/nchs/fastats/deaths.htm

188. Hagger-Johnson G, Gow AJ, Burley V, Greenwood D, Cade JE. Sitting Time, Fidgeting, and All-Cause Mortality in the UK Women's Cohort Study. Am J Prev Med. 2016;50(2):154-160. doi:10.1016/j.amepre.2015.06.025

189. Mustelin, L., Silventoinen, K., Pietiläinen, K. et al. Physical activity reduces the influence of genetic effects on BMI and waist circumference: a study in young adult twins. Int J Obes 33, 29–36 (2009). https://doi.org/10.1038/ijo.2008.258

152

190. https://pubmed.ncbi.nlm.nih.gov/19918249/)(Arsenault, B. J., Rana, J. S., Lemieux, I., Després, J.-P., Kastelein, J. J. P., Boekholdt, S. M., ... Khaw, K.-T. (2009). Physical inactivity, abdominal obesity and risk of coronary heart disease in apparently healthy men and women. International Journal of Obesity, 34(2), 340–347. doi: 10.1038/ijo.2009.229

191. https://pubmed.ncbi.nlm.nih.gov/20696950/)(Jacobs, E. J. (2010). Waist Circumference and All-Cause Mortality in a Large US Cohort. Archives of Internal Medicine, 170(15), 1293. doi: 10.1001/archinternmed.2010 .201

192. Nocon, M., Hiemann, T., Müller-Riemenschneider, F., Thalau, F., Roll, S., & Willich, S. N. (2008). Association of physical activity with all-cause and cardiovascular mortality: a systematic review and meta-analysis. European Journal of Cardiovascular Prevention & Rehabilitation, 15(3), 239–246. doi: 10.1097/hjr.0b013e3282f55e09

193. Hagger-Johnson, G., Gow, A. J., Burley, V., Greenwood, D., & Cade, J. E. (2016). Sitting Time, Fidgeting, and All-Cause Mortality in the UK Women's Cohort Study. American Journal of Preventive Medicine, 50(2), 154–160. doi: 10.1016/j.amepre.2015.06.025

194. Ohkawara K, Tanaka S, Miyachi M, Ishikawa-Takata K, Tabata I. A dose-response relation between aerobic exercise and visceral fat reduction: systematic review of clinical trials [published correction appears in Int J Obes (Lond). 2008 Feb;32(2):395]. Int J Obes (Lond). 2007;31(12):1786-1797. doi:10.1038/sj.ijo.0803683

195. Slentz, C. A., Aiken, L. B., Houmard, J. A., Bales, C. W., Johnson, J. L., Tanner, C. J., Duscha, B. D., & Kraus, W. E. (2005). Inactivity, exercise, and visceral fat. STRRIDE: a randomized, controlled study of exercise intensity and amount. Journal of Applied Physiology, 99(4), 1613–1618. https://doi.org/10.1152/japplphysiol.00124.2005

196. Santos-Baez LS, Ginsberg HN. Nonalcohol fatty liver disease: balancing supply and utilization of triglycerides. Curr Opin Lipidol. 2021 Jun 1;32(3):200-206. doi: 10.1097/MOL.0000000000000756. PMID: 33883445; PMCID: PMC8087156.

197. Fatty liver disease. (n.d.). UCLA Health. https://www.uclahealth.org/c omet/fatty-liver-disease

198. Johnson, N., Sachinwalla, T., Walton, D., Smith, K., Armstrong, A., Thompson, M., & George, J. (2009, June 15). Aerobic exercise training reduces hepatic and visceral lipids in obese individuals without weight loss. Retrieved June 05, 2020, from https://aasldpubs.onlinelibrary.wiley.com /doi/full/10.1002/hep.23129.

199. Arazi, Hamid & Farzaneh, Esmail & Gholamian, Samira. (2012). EFFECTS OF MORNING AEROBIC TRAINING ON LIPID PROFILE, BODY COMPOSITION, WHR AND VO 2max IN SEDENTARY OVERWEIGHT FEMALES. J Acta Kinesiologica. 1. 19-23.

200. U.S. Department of Health and Human Services. Physical Activity Guidelines for Americans, 2nd edition. Washington, DC: U.S. Department of Health and Human Services; 2018. https://health.gov/sites/def ault/files/2019-09/Physical_Activity_Guidelines_2nd_edition.pdf

201. Boutcher SH. High-intensity intermittent exercise and fat loss. J Obes. 2011;2011:868305. doi: 10.1155/2011/868305. Epub 2010 Nov 24. PMID: 21113312; PMCID: PMC2991639

202. Keating SE, Machan EA, O'Connor HT, Gerofi JA, Sainsbury A, Caterson ID, Johnson NA. Continuous exercise but not high intensity interval training improves fat distribution in overweight adults. J Obes. 2014;2014:834865. doi: 10.1155/2014/834865. Epub 2014 Jan 19. PMID: 24669314; PMCID: PMC3942093

203. Giannaki CD, Aphamis G, Sakkis P, Hadjicharalambous M. Eight weeks of a combination of high intensity interval training and conventional training reduce visceral adiposity and improve physical fitness: a group-based intervention. J Sports Med Phys Fitness 2016 April;56(4):483-90. https://www.minervamedica.it/en/journals/sports-med-physical-fitness/article.php?cod=R40Y2016N04A0483).

204. Kim TN, Park MS, Lim KI, Yang SJ, Yoo HJ, Kang HJ, Song W, Seo JA, Kim SG, Kim NH, Baik SH, Choi DS, Choi KM. Skeletal muscle mass to visceral fat area ratio is associated with metabolic syndrome and arterial stiffness: The Korean Sarcopenic Obesity Study (KSOS). Diabetes Res Clin Pract. 2011 Aug;93(2):285-291. doi: 10.1016/j.diabres.2011.06.01 3. Epub 2011 Jul 14. PMID: 21752483

154

205. Hart DW, Wolf SE, Zhang XJ, Chinkes DL, Buffalo MC, Matin SI, De-
bRoy MA, Wolfe RR, Herndon DN. Efficacy of a high-carbohydrate diet
in catabolic illness. Crit Care Med. 2001 Jul;29(7):1318-24. doi: 10.1097
/00003246-200107000-00004. PMID: 11445678. https://www.ncbi.nl
m.nih.gov/pubmed/11445678

206. Huang RY, Yang KC, Chang HH, Lee LT, Lu CW, Huang KC. The
Association between Total Protein and Vegetable Protein Intake and Low
Muscle Mass among the Community-Dwelling Elderly Population in
Northern Taiwan. Nutrients. 2016 Jun 17;8(6):373. doi: 10.3390/nu8
060373. PMID: 27322317; PMCID: PMC4924214. https://www.ncbi
.nlm.nih.gov/pubmed/27322317

207. Kinsey AW, Eddy WR, Madzima TA, et al. Influence of night-time protein
and carbohydrate intake on appetite and cardiometabolic risk in sedentary
overweight and obese women. British Journal of Nutrition.
2014;112(3):320-327.   doi:10.1017/S0007114514001068.
https://www.cambridge.org/core/journals/british-journal-of-nutrition/a
rticle/influence-of-nighttime-protein-and-carbohydrate-intake-on-appeti
te-and-cardiometabolic-risk-in-sedentary-overweight-and-obese-women/
5D66F9CB928136E64B73D848514F0C7C

208. Marci E Gluck, Colleen A Venti, Arline D Salbe, Jonathan
Krakoff, Nighttime eating: commonly observed and related to weight
gain in an inpatient food intake study, The American Journal
of Clinical Nutrition, Volume 88, Issue 4, October 2008, Pages
900–905, https://doi.org/10.1093/ajcn/88.4.900

209. Marci E Gluck, Colleen A Venti, Arline D Salbe, Jonathan
Krakoff, Nighttime eating: commonly observed and related to weight
gain in an inpatient food intake study, The American Journal
of Clinical Nutrition, Volume 88, Issue 4, October 2008, Pages
900–905, https://doi.org/10.1093/ajcn/88.4.900

210. Patterson, R. E., & Sears, D. D. (2017, July 17). Metabolic Effects of
Intermittent Fasting. Retrieved June 05, 2020, from https://www.annu
alreviews.org/doi/full/10.1146/annurev-nutr-071816-064634

211. Patterson, R. E., & Sears, D. D. (2017, July 17). Metabolic Effects of
Intermittent Fasting. Retrieved June 05, 2020, from https://www.annu
alreviews.org/doi/full/10.1146/annurev-nutr-071816-064634

212. Theorell-Haglöw, J., Berne, C., Janson, C., Sahlin, C., & Lindberg, E. (2010, May). Associations between short sleep duration and central obesity in women. Retrieved June 05, 2020, from https://www.ncbi.nlm.ni h.gov/pmc/articles/PMC2864874/

213. Theorell-Haglöw, J., Berne, C., Janson, C., Sahlin, C., & Lindberg, E. (2010, May). Associations between short sleep duration and central obesity in women. Retrieved June 05, 2020, from https://www.ncbi.nlm.ni h.gov/pmc/articles/PMC2864874/

214. Theorell-Haglöw, J., Berglund, L., Janson, C., & Lindberg, E. (2012, July 26). Sleep duration and central obesity in women – Differences between short sleepers and long sleepers. Retrieved June 05, 2020, from https:// www.sciencedirect.com/science/article/abs/pii/S1389945712002675

215. Kristen G. Hairston, MD, Michael Bryer-Ash, MD, Jill M. Norris, PhD, Steven Haffner, MD, Donald W. Bowden, PhD, Lynne E. Wagenknecht, DrPH, Sleep Duration and Five-Year Abdominal Fat Accumulation in a Minority Cohort: The IRAS Family Study, Sleep, Volume 33, Issue 3, March 2010, Pages 289–295, https://doi.org/10.1093/sleep/33.3.289

216. Ford, E., Li, C., Wheaton, A., Chapman, D., Perry, G., & Croft, J. (2013, October 15). Sleep duration and body mass index and waist circumference among Us adults. Retrieved June 05, 2020, from https://onlinelibrary.w iley.com/doi/full/10.1002/oby.20558

217. Clair, C., Chiolero, A., Faeh, D. et al. Dose-dependent positive association between cigarette smoking, abdominal obesity and body fat: cross-sectional data from a population-based survey. BMC Public Health 11, 23 (2011). https://doi.org/10.1186/1471-2458-11-23

218. Rose, K., Newman, B., Mayer-Davis, E., & Selby, J. (2012, September 06). Genetic and Behavioral Determinants of Waist-Hip Ratio and Waist Circumference in Women Twins. Retrieved June 05, 2020, from https:/ /onlinelibrary.wiley.com/doi/abs/10.1002/j.1550-8528.1998.tb00369.x

219. TS Han, FCH Bijnen, MEJ Lean, JC Seidell, Separate associations of waist and hip circumference with lifestyle factors, International Journal of Epidemiology, Volume 27, Issue 3, June 1998, Pages 422–430, https://doi.org/10.1093/ije/27.3.422

220. Adam D. Gepner, Megan E. Piper, Heather M. Johnson, Michael C. Fiore, Timothy B. Baker, James H. Stein. Effects of smoking and smoking cessation on lipids and lipoproteins: Outcomes from a randomized clinical trial. American Heart Journal, Volume 161, Issue 1, 2011, Pages 145-151, https://doi.org/10.1016/j.ahj.2010.09.023.

221. Johnson, H, Gossett, L, Piper, M. et al. Effects of Smoking and Smoking Cessation on Endothelial Function: 1-Year Outcomes From a Randomized Clinical Trial. J Am Coll Cardiol. 2010 May, 55 (18) 1988–1995.

222. Muniyappa R, Sable S, Ouwerkerk R, Mari A, Gharib AM, Walter M, Courville A, Hall G, Chen KY, Volkow ND, Kunos G, Huestis MA, Skarulis MC. Metabolic effects of chronic cannabis smoking. Diabetes Care. 2013 Aug;36(8):2415-22. doi: 10.2337/dc12-2303. Epub 2013 Mar 25. PMID: 23530011; PMCID: PMC3714514.

223. Al-Dabhani, K., Tsilidis, K., Murphy, N. et al. Prevalence of vitamin D deficiency and association with metabolic syndrome in a Qatari population. Nutr & Diabetes 7, e263 (2017). https://doi.org/10.1038/nutd.2017.14

224. Al-Mulhim NS, Eldin TG, Latif R, Al-Asoom LI, Al-Sunni A. Effects of vitamin D supplementation on anthropometric indices in vitamin D-deficient obese Saudi females; a randomized controlled trial. Saudi J Health Sci 2015;4:83-7.

225. Salehpour, A., Hosseinpanah, F., Shidfar, F. et al. A 12-week double-blind randomized clinical trial of vitamin D3supplementation on body fat mass in healthy overweight and obese women. Nutr J 11, 78 (2012). https://doi.org/10.1186/1475-2891-11-78

226. Barchetta I, Angelico F, Del Ben M, Baroni MG, Pozzilli P, Morini S, Cavallo MG. Strong association between non alcoholic fatty liver disease (NAFLD) and low 25(OH) vitamin D levels in an adult population with normal serum liver enzymes. BMC Med. 2011 Jul 12;9:85. doi: 10.1186/1741-7015-9-85. PMID: 21749681; PMCID: PMC3148980.

227. Cannell, J., Hollis, B.W., Sorenson, M.B., Taft, T.N., & Anderson, J.J. (2009). Athletic performance and vitamin D. Medicine and science in sports and exercise, 41 5, 1102-10. https://www.semanticscholar.org/paper/Athletic-performance-and-vita min-D.-Cannell-Hollis/61641c9d01a15a5d2c2654420b94a2cf61207bd 3?p2df

228. Carrillo, A. E., Flynn, M. G., Pinkston, C., Markofski, M. M., Jiang, Y., Donkin, S. S., & Teegarden, D. (2013). Impact of vitamin D supplementation during a resistance training intervention on body composition, muscle function, and glucose tolerance in overweight and obese adults. Clinical Nutrition, 32(3), 375–381. https://doi.org/10.1016/j.clnu.201 2.08.014

229. Nimitphong H, Samittarucksa R, Saetung S, Bhirommuang N, Chailurkit LO, Ongphiphadhanakul B. The Effect of Vitamin D Supplementation on Metabolic Phenotypes in Thais with Prediabetes. J Med Assoc Thai. 2015 Dec;98(12):1169-78. PMID: 27004301.

230. Nimitphong H, Samittarucksa R, Saetung S, Bhirommuang N, Chailurkit LO, Ongphiphadhanakul B. The Effect of Vitamin D Supplementation on Metabolic Phenotypes in Thais with Prediabetes. J Med Assoc Thai. 2015 Dec;98(12):1169-78. PMID: 27004301.

231. Nagatomo A, Nishida N, Fukuhara I, Noro A, Kozai Y, Sato H, Matsuura Y. Daily intake of rosehip extract decreases abdominal visceral fat in preobese subjects: a randomized, double-blind, placebo-controlled clinical trial. Diabetes Metab Syndr Obes. 2015 Mar 6;8:147-56. doi: 10.2147/ DMSO.S78623. PMID: 25834460; PMCID: PMC4358417. https://w ww.ncbi.nlm.nih.gov/pmc/articles/PMC4358417/

232. Wan-Loy C, Siew-Moi P. Marine Algae as a Potential Source for Anti-Obesity Agents. Mar Drugs. 2016 Dec 7;14(12):222. doi: 10.3390 /md14120222. PMID: 27941599; PMCID: PMC5192459. https://ww w.ncbi.nlm.nih.gov/pmc/articles/PMC5192459/

233. Xi Ding, Yang Zhao, Chun-Ying Zhu, Li-Ping Wu, Yue Wang, Zhao-Yi Peng, Cuomu Deji, Feng-Yi Zhao, Bing-Yin Shi, The association between subclinical hypothyroidism and metabolic syndrome: an update meta-analysis of observational studies, Endocrine Journal, 2021, Volume 68, Issue 9, Pages 1043-1056, Released on J-STAGE September 28, 2021, Advance online publication April 21, 2021, Online ISSN 1348-4540, Print ISSN 0918-8959, https://doi.org/10.1507/endocrj.EJ20-0796, https://www.jstage.jst.go.jp/article/endocrj/68/9/68_EJ20-0796/_article/-char/en

234. Combet E, Ma ZF, Cousins F, Thompson B, Lean ME. Low-level seaweed supplementation improves iodine status in iodine-insufficient women. Br J Nutr. 2014 Sep 14;112(5):753-61. doi: 10.1017/S0007114514001573. Epub 2014 Jul 9. PMID: 25006699. https://pubmed.ncbi.nlm.nih.gov/25006699/

235. Teas, J., Baldeón, M. E., Chiriboga, D. E., Davis, J. R., Sarriés, A. J., & Braverman, L. E. (2009). Could Dietary Seaweed Reverse the Metabolic Syndrome?. Asia Pacific Journal of Clinical Nutrition, 18(2), 145-154. https://doi.org/10.6133/apjcn.2009.18.2.01

236. Jane Teas, Thomas G. Hurley, James R. Hebert, Adrian A. Franke, Daniel W. Sepkovic, Mindy S. Kurzer. Dietary Seaweed Modifies Estrogen and Phytoestrogen Metabolism in Healthy Postmenopausal Women12. The Journal of Nutrition, Volume 139, Issue 5, 2009, Pages 939-944, ISSN 0022-3166, https://doi.org/10.3945/jn.108.100834.

237. Stoddard II FR, Brooks AD, Eskin BA, Johannes GJ. Iodine Alters Gene Expression in the MCF7 Breast Cancer Cell Line: Evidence for an Anti-Estrogen Effect of Iodine. Int J Med Sci 2008; 5(4):189-196. doi:10.7150/ijms.5.189. https://www.medsci.org/v05p0189.htm

238. Hitoe, S., & Shimoda, H. (2017). Seaweed fucoxanthin supplementation improves obesity parameters in mild obese Japanese subjects. Functional Foods in Health and Disease, 7(4), 246. https://doi.org/10.31989/ffhd.v7i4.333

239. Teas, J., Baldeón, M. E., Chiriboga, D. E., Davis, J. R., Sarriés, A. J., & Braverman, L. E. (2009). Could Dietary Seaweed Reverse the Metabolic Syndrome?. Asia Pacific Journal of Clinical Nutrition, 18(2), 145-154. https://doi.org/10.6133/apjcn.2009.18.2.01

240. Yin, J., Wang, C., Shao, Q., Qu, D., Song, Z., Shan, P., Zhang, T., Xu, J., Qin, L., Zhang, S., & Huang, J. (2014). Relationship between the Prevalence of Thyroid Nodules and Metabolic Syndrome in the Iodine-Adequate Area of Hangzhou, China: A Cross-Sectional and Cohort Study. International Journal of Endocrinology, 2014, 1–7. https://doi.org/10.1155/2014/675796

241. Kitahara CM, Platz EA, Ladenson PW, Mondul AM, Menke A, de González AB (2012) Body Fatness and Markers of Thyroid Function among U.S. Men and Women. PLoS ONE 7(4): e34979. https://doi.org/10.1371/journal.pone.0034979

242. Meissner HO, Kedzia B, Mrozikiewicz PM, Mscisz A. Short and long-term physiological responses of male and female rats to two dietary levels of pre-gelatinized maca (lepidium peruvianum chacon). Int J Biomed Sci. 2006 Feb;2(1):13-28. PMID: 23674962; PMCID: PMC3614567.

243. Abidov M, Ramazanov Z, Seifulla R, Grachev S. The effects of Xanthigen in the weight management of obese premenopausal women with non-alcoholic fatty liver disease and normal liver fat. Diabetes Obes Metab. 2010 Jan;12(1):72-81. doi: 10.1111/j.1463-1326.2009.01132.x. Epub 2009 Oct 13. PMID: 19840063.

244. Kim KM, Kim SM, Cho DY, Park SJ, Joo NS. The Effect of Xanthigen on the Expression of Brown Adipose Tissue Assessed by ^{18}F-FDG PET. Yonsei Med J. 2016 Jul;57(4):1038-1041. doi: 10.3349/ymj.2016.57.4.1038. PMID: 27189303; PMCID: PMC4951448.https://www.ncbi.nlm.nih.gov/pmc/articles/PMC4951448/

245. Genta S, Cabrera W, Habib N, Pons J, Carillo IM, Grau A, Sánchez S. Yacon syrup: beneficial effects on obesity and insulin resistance in humans. Clin Nutr. 2009 Apr;28(2):182-7. doi: 10.1016/j.clnu.2009.01.013. Epub 2009 Feb 28. PMID: 19254816.

246. Genta S, Cabrera W, Habib N, Pons J, Carillo IM, Grau A, Sánchez S. Yacon syrup: beneficial effects on obesity and insulin resistance in humans. Clin Nutr. 2009 Apr;28(2):182-7. doi: 10.1016/j.clnu.2009.01.013. Epub 2009 Feb 28. PMID: 19254816.

247. Joseph Jewel Ann, Akkermans Simen, Nimmegeers Philippe, Van Impe Jan F. M. Bioproduction of the Recombinant Sweet Protein Thaumatin: Current State of the Art and Perspectives. Frontiers in Microbiology. Volume 10, 2019. https://www.frontiersin.org/articles/10.3389/fmicb.201 9.00695.

248. Kubota K, Sumi S, Tojo H, Sumi-Inoue Y, I-Chin H, Oi Y, Fujita H, Urata H. Improvements of mean body mass index and body weight in preobese and overweight Japanese adults with black Chinese tea (Pu-Erh) water extract. Nutr Res. 2011 Jun;31(6):421-8. doi: 10.1016/j.nutres.20 11.05.004. Epub 2011 Jun 17. Erratum in: Nutr Res. 2012 Jun;32(6):470. PMID: 21745623.

249. Chu SL, Fu H, Yang JX, Liu GX, Dou P, Zhang L, Tu PF, Wang XM. A randomized double-blind placebo-controlled study of Pu'er tea extract on the regulation of metabolic syndrome. Chin J Integr Med. 2011 Jul;17(7):492-8. doi: 10.1007/s11655-011-0781-4. Epub 2011 Jul 3. PMID: 21725873.

250. Lehtonen HM, Suomela JP, Tahvonen R, Yang B, Venojärvi M, Viikari J, Kallio H. Different berries and berry fractions have various but slightly positive effects on the associated variables of metabolic diseases on overweight and obese women. Eur J Clin Nutr. 2011 Mar;65(3):394-401. doi: 10.1038/ejcn.2010.268. Epub 2011 Jan 12. PMID: 21224867.

251. Johnston CS, Beezhold BL, Mostow B, Swan PD. Plasma vitamin C is inversely related to body mass index and waist circumference but not to plasma adiponectin in nonsmoking adults. J Nutr. 2007 Jul;137(7):1757-62. doi: 10.1093/jn/137.7.1757. PMID: 17585027.

252. Harunobu Amagase & Dwight M Nance (2011) Lycium barbarum Increases Caloric Expenditure and Decreases Waist Circumference in Healthy Overweight Men and Women: Pilot Study, Journal of the American College of Nutrition, 30:5, 304-309, DOI: 10.1080/07315724.2011.10719973

253. Wang H, Wen Y, Du Y, Yan X, Guo H, Rycroft JA, Boon N, Kovacs EM, Mela DJ. Effects of catechin enriched green tea on body composition. Obesity (Silver Spring). 2010 Apr;18(4):773-9. doi: 10.1038/oby.2009.256. Epub 2009 Aug 13. PMID: 19680234.

254. J. Münzker, D. Hofer, C. Trummer, M. Ulbing, A. Harger, T. Pieber, L. Owen, B. Keevil, G. Brabant, E. Lerchbaum, B. Obermayer-Pietsch, Testosterone to Dihydrotestosterone Ratio as a New Biomarker for an Adverse Metabolic Phenotype in the Polycystic Ovary Syndrome, The Journal of Clinical Endocrinology & Metabolism, Volume 100, Issue 2, 1 February 2015, Pages 653–660, https://doi.org/10.1210/jc.2014-2523

255. Nelson Prager, Karen Bickett, Nita French, and Geno Marcovici. A Randomized, Double-Blind, Placebo-Controlled Trial to Determine the Effectiveness of Botanically Derived Inhibitors of 5-α-Reductase in the Treatment of Androgenetic Alopecia. The Journal of Alternative and Complementary Medicine 2002 8:2, 143-152

256. J. Münzker, D. Hofer, C. Trummer, M. Ulbing, A. Harger, T. Pieber, L. Owen, B. Keevil, G. Brabant, E. Lerchbaum, B. Obermayer-Pietsch, Testosterone to Dihydrotestosterone Ratio as a New Biomarker for an Adverse Metabolic Phenotype in the Polycystic Ovary Syndrome, The Journal of Clinical Endocrinology & Metabolism, Volume 100, Issue 2, 1 February 2015, Pages 653–660, https://doi.org/10.1210/jc.2014-2523

257. Ovarian overproduction of androgens: MedlinePlus Medical Encyclopedia. (n.d.). https://medlineplus.gov/ency/article/001165.htm

258. Waetzig, G. H., Rosenstiel, P., Arlt, A., Till, A., Bräutigam, K., Schäfer, H., Rose-John, S., Seegert, D., & Schreiber, S. (2004). Soluble tumor necrosis factor (TNF) receptor-1 induces apoptosis via reverse TNF signaling and autocrine transforming growth factor-β1. The FASEB Journal, 19(1), 91–93. https://doi.org/10.1096/fj.04-2073fje

259. Pirillo A, Catapano AL. Berberine, a plant alkaloid with lipid- and glucose-lowering properties: From in vitro evidence to clinical studies. Atherosclerosis. 2015 Dec;243(2):449-61. doi: 10.1016/j.atherosclerosis.2015.09.032. Epub 2015 Sep 30. PMID: 26520899. https://pubmed.ncbi.nlm.nih.gov/26520899/

260. Xiong P, Niu L, Talaei S, Kord-Varkaneh H, Clark CCT, Găman MA, Rahmani J, Dorosti M, Mousavi SM, Zarezadeh M, Taghizade-Bilondi H, Zhang J. The effect of berberine supplementation on obesity indices: A dose- response meta-analysis and systematic review of randomized controlled trials. Complement Ther Clin Pract. 2020 May;39:101113. doi: 10.1016/j.ctcp.2020.101113. Epub 2020 Feb 1. PMID: 32379652. http s://pubmed.ncbi.nlm.nih.gov/32379652/

261. Yadav, Dharmendra. Bharitkar, Yogesh. Chatterjee, Kasturi. Ghosh, Monisangar, Mondal, Nirup. Swarnakar, Snehasikta. Importance of Neem Leaf: An Insight Into its role in combating diseases. Indian Journal of Experimental Biology. Vol. 54, November 2016, pp. 708-718. https://nopr.niscpr.res.in/bitstream/123456789/36892/1/IJ EB%2054%2811%29%20708-718.pdf

262. Batra N, Kumar VE, Nambiar R, De Souza C, Yuen A, Le U, Verma R, Ghosh PM, Vinall RL. Exploring the therapeutic potential of Neem (Azadirachta Indica) for the treatment of prostate cancer: a literature review. Ann Transl Med. 2022 Jul;10(13):754. doi: 10.21037/atm-22-94. PMID: 35957716; PMCID: PMC9358515. https://pubmed.ncbi.nlm. nih.gov/35957716/

263. Asghar, H. A., Abbas, S. Q., Arshad, M., Jabin, A., Usman, B., Aslam, M., & Asghar, A. (2022). Therapeutic Potential of Azadirachta indica (Neem)-A Comprehensive Review. Scholars International Journal of Traditional and Complementary Medicine, 5(3), 47–64. https://doi.org/10 .36348/sijtcm.2022.v05i03.001

264. Verdam, F. J., Fuentes, S., De Jonge, C., Zoetendal, E. G., Erbil, R., Greve, J., Buurman, W. A., De Vos, W. M., & Rensen, S. S. (2013). Human intestinal microbiota composition is associated with local and systemic inflammation in obesity. Obesity, 21(12). https://doi.org/10.1002/oby. 20466

265. Verdam, F. J., Fuentes, S., De Jonge, C., Zoetendal, E. G., Erbil, R., Greve, J., Buurman, W. A., De Vos, W. M., & Rensen, S. S. (2013). Human intestinal microbiota composition is associated with local and systemic inflammation in obesity. Obesity, 21(12). https://doi.org/10.1002/oby. 20466

266. Verdam, F. J., Fuentes, S., De Jonge, C., Zoetendal, E. G., Erbil, R., Greve, J., Buurman, W. A., De Vos, W. M., & Rensen, S. S. (2013). Human intestinal microbiota composition is associated with local and systemic inflammation in obesity. Obesity, 21(12). https://doi.org/10.1002/oby.20466

267. Machate, D. J., Figueiredo, P. G., Marcelino, G., De Cássia Avellaneda Guimarães, R., Hiane, P. A., Bogo, D., Zorgetto-Pinheiro, V. A., De Oliveira, L. C. S., & Pott, A. (2020). Fatty acid diets: regulation of gut microbiota composition and obesity and its related metabolic dysbiosis. International Journal of Molecular Sciences, 21(11), 4093. https://doi.org/10.3390/ijms21114093

268. Yin XQ, An YX, Yu CG, Ke J, Zhao D, Yu K. The Association Between Fecal Short-Chain Fatty Acids, Gut Microbiota, and Visceral Fat in Monozygotic Twin Pairs. Diabetes Metab Syndr Obes. 2022 Feb 5;15:359-368. doi: 10.2147/DMSO.S338113. PMID: 35153497; PMCID: PMC8828081. www.ncbi.nlm.nih.gov/pmc/articles/PMC8828081/

269. Pinart, M., Dötsch, A., Schlicht, K., Laudes, M., Bouwman, J., Forslund, K., Pischon, T., & Nimptsch, K. (2021). Gut Microbiome Composition in Obese and Non-Obese Persons: A Systematic Review and Meta-Analysis. Nutrients, 14(1), 12. https://doi.org/10.3390/nu14010012

270. Sheng, Y., Liu, J., Zheng, S., Liang, F., Luo, Y., Huang, K., Xu, W., & He, X. (2019). Mulberry leaves ameliorate obesity through enhancing brown adipose tissue activity and modulating gut microbiota. Food & Function, 10(8), 4771–4781. https://doi.org/10.1039/c9fo00883g

271. Zellner T, Prasa D, Färber E, Hoffmann-Walbeck P, Genser D, Eyer F. The Use of Activated Charcoal to Treat Intoxications. Dtsch Arztebl Int. 2019 May 3;116(18):311-317. doi: 10.3238/arztebl.2019.0311. PMID: 31219028; PMCID: PMC6620762. https://www.ncbi.nlm.nih.gov/pmc/articles/PMC6620762/

272. Virginia Tech. https://ext.vt.edu/natural-resources/charcoal/charcoalmaking.html#:~:text=Introduction%3A,gives%20off%20heat%20once%20started.

273. Rahman MM, Adil M, Yusof AM, Kamaruzzaman YB, Ansary RH. Removal of Heavy Metal Ions with Acid Activated Carbons Derived from Oil Palm and Coconut Shells. Materials (Basel). 2014 May 7;7(5):3634-3650. doi: 10.3390/ma7053634. PMID: 28788640; PMCID: PMC5453229. https://www.ncbi.nlm.nih.gov/pmc/articles/PMC5453229/

274. Zhang X, Diao P, Yokoyama H, Inoue Y, Tanabe K, Wang X, Hayashi C, Yokoyama T, Zhang Z, Hu X, Nakajima T, Kimura T, Nakayama J, Nakamuta M, Tanaka N. Acidic Activated Charcoal Prevents Obesity and Insulin Resistance in High-Fat Diet-Fed Mice. Front Nutr. 2022 May 12;9:852767. doi: 10.3389/fnut.2022.852767. PMID: 35634388; PMCID: PMC9134190. https://www.ncbi.nlm.nih.gov/pmc/articles/PMC9134190/

275. Sugimoto K, Shinagawa T, Kuroki K, Toma S, Hosomi R, Yoshida M, Fukunaga K. Dietary Bamboo Charcoal Decreased Visceral Adipose Tissue Weight by Enhancing Fecal Lipid Excretions in Mice with High-Fat Diet-Induced Obesity. Prev Nutr Food Sci. 2023 Sep 30;28(3):246-254. doi: 10.3746/pnf.2023.28.3.246. PMID: 37842254; PMCID: PMC10567601. https://www.ncbi.nlm.nih.gov/pmc/articles/PMC10567601/

276. Neuvonen PJ, Kuusisto P, Vapaatalo H, Manninen V. Activated charcoal in the treatment of hypercholesterolaemia: dose-response relationships and comparison with cholestyramine. Eur J Clin Pharmacol. 1989;37(3):225-30. doi: 10.1007/BF00679774. PMID: 2612535. https://pubmed.ncbi.nlm.nih.gov/2612535/

277. Petre, A., MS, RD (NL). (2023, February 23). What Is Activated Charcoal? Benefits and Uses (G. Dunsmith, Ed.). Healthline. https://www.healthline.com/nutrition/activated-charcoal

278. Naka, K., Watarai, S., Tana, Inoue, K., Kodama, Y., Oguma, K., Yasuda, T., & Kodama, H. (2001). Adsorption Effect of Activated Charcoal on Enterohemorrhagic Escherichia coli. Journal of Veterinary Medical Science, 63(3), 281–285. https://doi.org/10.1292/jvms.63.281

279. Rahman MM, Alam MN, Ulla A, Sumi FA, Subhan N, Khan T, Sikder B, Hossain H, Reza HM, Alam MA. Cardamom powder supplementation prevents obesity, improves glucose intolerance, inflammation and oxidative stress in liver of high carbohydrate high fat diet induced obese rats. Lipids Health Dis. 2017 Aug 14;16(1):151. doi: 10.1186/s12944-017-0 539-x. PMID: 28806968; PMCID: PMC5557534. https://pubmed.ncb i.nlm.nih.gov/28806968/

280. Kazemi S, Yaghooblou F, Siassi F, Rahimi Foroushani A, Ghavipour M, Koohdani F, Sotoudeh G. Cardamom supplementation improves inflammatory and oxidative stress biomarkers in hyperlipidemic, overweight, and obese pre-diabetic women: a randomized double-blind clinical trial. J Sci Food Agric. 2017 Dec;97(15):5296-5301. doi: 10.1002/jsfa.8414. Epub 2017 Jul 17. PMID: 28480505.https://pubmed.ncbi.nlm.nih.gov/2848 0505/

281. Cheshmeh S, Ghayyem M, Khamooshi F, Heidarzadeh-Esfahani N, Rahmani N, Hojati N, Mosaieby E, Moradi S, Pasdar Y. Green cardamom plus low-calorie diet can decrease the expression of inflammatory genes among obese women with polycystic ovary syndrome: a double-blind randomized clinical trial. Eat Weight Disord. 2022 Mar;27(2):821-830. doi: 10.1007 /s40519-021-01223-3. Epub 2021 May 31. PMID: 34057705; PMCID: PMC8166375.https://pubmed.ncbi.nlm.nih.gov/34057705/

282. Rahimlou, M., Yari, Z., Rayyani, E. et al. Effects of ginger supplementation on anthropometric, glycemic and metabolic parameters in subjects with metabolic syndrome: A randomized, double-blind, placebo-controlled study. J Diabetes Metab Disord 18, 119–125 (2019). https://do i.org/10.1007/s40200-019-00397-z

283. Najmeh Maharlouei, Reza Tabrizi, Kamran B. Lankarani, Abbas Rezaianzadeh, Maryam Akbari, Fariba Kolahdooz, Maryam Rahimi, Fariba Keneshlou & Zatollah Asemi (2019) The effects of ginger intake on weight loss and metabolic profiles among overweight and obese subjects: A systematic review and meta-analysis of randomized controlled trials, Critical Reviews in Food Science and Nutrition, 59:11, 1753-1766, DOI: 10.1080/10408398.2018.1427044https://www.tandfonline.com/doi/abs/10.1080/10408398.2018.1427044

166

284. Wang, J., Wang, P., Li, D. et al. Beneficial effects of ginger on prevention of obesity through modulation of gut microbiota in mice. Eur J Nutr 59, 699–718 (2020). https://doi.org/10.1007/s00394-019-01938-1

285. Yin XQ, An YX, Yu CG, Ke J, Zhao D, Yu K. The Association Between Fecal Short-Chain Fatty Acids, Gut Microbiota, and Visceral Fat in Monozygotic Twin Pairs. Diabetes Metab Syndr Obes. 2022 Feb 5;15:359-368. doi: 10.2147/DMSO.S338113. PMID: 35153497; PMCID: PMC8828081. https://www.ncbi.nlm.nih.gov/pmc/articles/PMC8828081/

286. Razmpoosh, E., Safi, S., Nadjarzadeh, A. et al. The effect of Nigella sativa supplementation on cardiovascular risk factors in obese and overweight women: a crossover, double-blind, placebo-controlled randomized clinical trial. Eur J Nutr 60, 1863–1874 (2021). https://doi.org/10.1007/s00394-020-02374-2

287. Farzaneh E, Nia FR, Mehrtash M, Mirmoeini FS, Jalilvand M. The Effects of 8-week Nigella sativa Supplementation and Aerobic Training on Lipid Profile and VO2 max in Sedentary Overweight Females. Int J Prev Med. 2014 Feb;5(2):210-6. PMID: 24627749; PMCID: PMC3950745. https://www.ncbi.nlm.nih.gov/pmc/articles/PMC3950745/

288. Al Asoom L. Is Nigella sativa an Effective Bodyweight Lowering Agent and a Mitigator of Obesity Risk? A Literature Review. Vasc Health Risk Manag. 2022 Jul 12;18:495-505. doi: 10.2147/VHRM.S373702. PMID: 35855753; PMCID: PMC9288173. https://www.ncbi.nlm.nih.gov/pmc/articles/PMC9288173/

289. Nazli Namazi, Bagher Larijani, Mohammad Hossein Ayati, Mohammad Abdollahi. The effects of Nigella sativa L. on obesity: A systematic review and meta-analysis. Journal of Ethnopharmacology, Volume 219, 2018, Pages 173-181. https://doi.org/10.1016/j.jep.2018.03.001.

290. Sara Safi, Elham Razmpoosh, Hossien Fallahzadeh, Mahta Mazaheri, Nooshin Abdollahi, Majid Nazari, Azadeh Nadjarzadeh, Amin Salehi-Abargouei. The effect of Nigella sativa on appetite, anthropometric and body composition indices among overweight and obese women: A crossover, double-blind, placebo-controlled, randomized clinical trial. Complementary Therapies in Medicine, Volume 57, 2021, 102653, ISSN 0965-2299. https://doi.org/10.1016/j.ctim.2020.102653.

291. Dehzad, M. J., Ghalandari, H., Nouri, M., & Askarpour, M. (2023). Effects of curcumin/turmeric supplementation on obesity indices and adipokines in adults: A grade-assessed systematic review and dose–response meta-analysis of randomized controlled trials. Phytotherapy Research, 37(4), 1703–1728. https://doi.org/10.1002/ptr.7800

292. Safari, Z., Bagherniya, M., Askari, G., Sathyapalan, T., & Sahebkar, A. (2021). The effect of curcumin supplementation on anthropometric indices in overweight and obese individuals: a systematic review of randomized controlled trials. In Advances in Experimental Medicine and Biology (pp. 121–137). https://doi.org/10.1007/978-3-030-56153-6_7

293. Lee, C. H., Kim, A., Pyun, C., Fukushima, M., & Han, K. (2013). Turmeric (Curcuma longa) whole powder reduces accumulation of visceral fat mass and increases hepatic oxidative stress in rats fed a high-fat diet. Food Science and Biotechnology, 23(1), 261–267. https://doi.org/10.1007/s10068-014-0036-1

294. Javad Heshmati, Ashraf Moini, Mahdi Sepidarkish, Mojgan Morvaridzadeh, Masoud Salehi, Andriko Palmowski, Maryam Farid Mojtahedi, Farzad Shidfar. Effects of curcumin supplementation on blood glucose, insulin resistance and androgens in patients with polycystic ovary syndrome: A randomized double-blind placebo-controlled clinical trial. Phytomedicine. Volume 80, 2021, 153395. https://doi.org/10.1016/j.phymed.2020.153395.

295. Alvord, M., Kelly, J., Tovian, S., Davidson, K., & McGuiness, K. Understanding Chronic Stress. Retrieved from https://www.apa.org/helpcenter/understanding-chronic-stress. Stress won't go away? Maybe you are suffering from chronic stress. (2022, November 1). https://www.apa.org. https://www.apa.org/helpcenter/understanding-chronic-stress

296. Stellar JE, John-Henderson N, Anderson CL, Gordon AM, McNeil GD, Keltner D. Positive affect and markers of inflammation: discrete positive emotions predict lower levels of inflammatory cytokines. Emotion. 2015 Apr;15(2):129-33. doi: 10.1037/emo0000033. Epub 2015 Jan 19. PMID: 25603133.

297. Stachowicz, M., Lebiedzińska, A. The effect of diet components on the level of cortisol. Eur Food Res Technol 242, 2001–2009 (2016). https://doi.org/10.1007/s00217-016-2772-3

298. Stachowicz, M., & Lebiedzińska, A. (2016). The effect of diet components on the level of cortisol. European Food Research and Technology, 242(12), 2001–2009. doi: 10.1007/s00217-016-2772-3

299. Ong AD, Benson L, Zautra AJ, Ram N. Emodiversity and biomarkers of inflammation. Emotion. 2018 Feb;18(1):3-14. doi: 10.1037/emo0000343. Epub 2017 Jun 22. PMID: 28639792; PMCID: PMC6145448. https://pubmed.ncbi.nlm.nih.gov/28639792/

300. Maydych, V. (2019). The Interplay Between Stress, Inflammation, and Emotional Attention: Relevance for Depression. Frontiers in Neuroscience, 13(384). doi: 10.3389/fnins.2019.00384

301. Trudel-Fitzgerald, C., Qureshi, F., Appleton, A. A., & Kubzansky, L. D. (2017). A healthy mix of emotions: underlying biological pathways linking emotions to physical health. Current Opinion in Behavioral Sciences, 15, 16–21. doi: 10.1016/j.cobeha.2017.05.003

302. Moons, W. G., Eisenberger, N. I., & Taylor, S. E. (2009). Anger and fear responses to stress have different biological profiles. Brain, Behavior, and Immunity, 24(2), 215–219. doi: 10.1016/j.bbi.2009.08.009.

303. Stellar JE, John-Henderson N, Anderson CL, Gordon AM, McNeil GD, Keltner D. Positive affect and markers of inflammation: discrete positive emotions predict lower levels of inflammatory cytokines. Emotion. 2015 Apr;15(2):129-33. doi: 10.1037/emo0000033. Epub 2015 Jan 19. PMID: 25603133.

304. Stellar JE, John-Henderson N, Anderson CL, Gordon AM, McNeil GD, Keltner D. Positive affect and markers of inflammation: discrete positive emotions predict lower levels of inflammatory cytokines. Emotion. 2015 Apr;15(2):129-33. doi: 10.1037/emo0000033. Epub 2015 Jan 19. PMID: 25603133.

305. Sheldon, K.M., Abad, N., Ferguson, Y. et al. Persistent pursuit of need-satisfying goals leads to increased happiness: A 6-month experimental longitudinal study. Motiv Emot 34, 39–48 (2010). https://doi.org/10.1007/s11031-009-9153-1 https://link.springer.com/article/10.1007/s11031-009-9153-1

www.ingramcontent.com/pod-product-compliance
Lightning Source LLC
Chambersburg PA
CBHW070806280326
41934CB00012B/3074